28 Day Chair Yoga for Seniors

Stay Active, Relaxed, and Healthy with Gentle Chair Yoga Exercises

Anna Caine

The information herein is solely offered for informational purposes and is universal. The presentation of the information is without a contract or any guarantee assurance.

The trademarks used are without any consent, and the trademark publication is without permission or backing by the trademark owner. All trademarks and brands within this book are for clarifying purposes only and are owned by the owners, not affiliated with this document.

Table of Contents

Get Updates and Bonuses

Introduction

When we live in a world that seems to move at a faster pace with each passing day, and when time becomes the most elusive item we own, it is not unexpected that we regularly neglect to take care of ourselves. In fact, it is not surprising at all. Due to the fact that we are caught up in the whirlwind of responsibilities, which includes juggling a work, family, and a plethora of other commitments from time to time, there is very little room for us to take care of our own health. Nevertheless, in the middle of all this chaos, there is one set of individuals who typically suffer the most from neglect: the elderly among us. They are the ones who are most likely to be neglected.

Take the following example into consideration: You find yourself standing in front of the mirror, staring at the reflection of a person whom you hardly know anymore. It is yet another normal day, and you find yourself in this situation. In addition to telling the stories of a life well-lived, the lines that have been etched into your skin also carry the message that time has taken its toll on your body. This makes the lines a visual representation of the passage of time. Perhaps you wake up with a tiny increase in the pain that you experience in your joints, or perhaps the stiffness that you experience in your muscles acts as a constant reminder of the fact that you are progressively becoming older. Both of these symptoms could be a sign that you are becoming older. It is obvious that becoming older is accompanied by a certain number of challenges, such as those that are both physical and emotional in nature. This is the case regardless of the circumstances that one is in.

However, here's the thing: becoming older does not necessarily mean that one's quality of life will deteriorate. This is something that should be mentioned. To be more precise, the opposite is true in every respect. Regardless of your age or the physical limitations you may be facing, you have the capacity to recover control over your health and well-being if you have access to the necessary resources and knowledge. This is true regardless of whether you are physically disabled or not. It is precisely in this context that this book comes into their own.

We would like to take this time to extend a warm welcome to you as you enter "28 Day Chair Yoga For Seniors," your comprehensive guide to releasing the transformative power of yoga from the comfort of your own lounge chair. Now, before you dismiss the idea that yoga is something that is just for the young and flexible, allow me to reassure you that this practice was deliberate designed with the intention of meeting the requirements of senior persons in order to meet their demands. It is no longer necessary to struggle to keep up with the pace of a conventional yoga practice or to distort your body into positions that resemble pretzels. These days are long gone. As an alternative, we would like to give to you an invitation to take a seat, make yourself comfortable in your chair, and go on a trip that will lead to improved health, vitality, and mental calm. We hope that you will accept this invitation.

Now, you might be wondering, why yoga? Where does this time-honored practice stand in comparison to the myriad other forms of physical activity that are competing for your attention? It takes a holistic approach to wellbeing, which means that it not only addresses the physical aspects of health but also nurtures the mind-body connection, which is at the center of our well-being. This is the answer. The practice of yoga provides a means to achieve better flexibility, strength, and resilience, all of which are critical components of healthy aging. Yoga is accomplished via the use of gentle stretches, focused breathing, and relaxation techniques.

Throughout the course of reading this book, you will come across a plethora of advantages that are waiting for you. Every new day brings with it new potential for personal development and healing, including the reduction of pain and tension, as well as improvements in mobility and balance. And perhaps even more crucially, you will discover a sense of community and support that is unlike anything else you've ever experienced. You will be reminded that you are not alone in your problems as you embark on this journey alongside other seniors. You will also be reminded that there is power in shared experience and strength in solidarity.

In light of this, what can you anticipate gaining from reading these pages? We will lead you through a series of gentle yoga practices that are meant to meet you precisely where you are at this moment in time throughout the course of a period of 28 days. Each and every session is carefully developed to cater to your specific requirements and capabilities, regardless of whether you are a complete novice or an experienced practitioner. For visual learners, we've included easy-to-follow video demonstrations that you can access by scanning the QR code provided. This ensures you perform each exercise correctly and safely. In this course, you will learn about a number of practices that are designed to improve both your physical and mental well-being. These techniques include guided meditations and seated stretches.

However, in addition to the postures themselves, this book is also a guide to developing a more profound sense of self-awareness and compassion. Through the use of guided mindfulness exercises and reflective writing prompts, you will acquire the ability to listen to the information that your body has to provide and to respect its intrinsic capability for healing. By engaging in such activities, you will not only improve your body, but you will also create a greater sense of resilience in the face of the obstacles that are unavoidable in life.

It's possible that you're wondering why you should place your trust in me to guide you further on this journey at this moment in time. It is my pleasure to make a presentation on the topic of yoga for senior persons. To what extent do I possess credentials? To tell you the truth, I have been in the exact same situation as you are right now. The discomfort that I feel in my joints and the stiffness that I feel in my muscles are both things that I have experienced. Overcoming the challenges that come with getting older is something that I have personally experienced, and I have discovered that yoga has the capacity to change and assist me in overcoming these challenges. The great impact that this practice can have on the lives of people who are similar to you is something that I have witnessed myself as a yoga instructor who is certified and has years of experience working with senior persons.

In addition to that, however, I am really excited about the prospect of teaching yoga to other people and inspiring senior folks to take responsibility for their own health and well-being. I am extremely enthused about the thought of doing both of these things. I have no doubt in my mind that this method has the potential to bring about a transformation, and I am committed to providing you with assistance during each and every stage of the process.

As a result, if you are willing to embark on a journey that will result in enhanced physical health, vitality, and mental peace, then I would like to extend an invitation to you to join me on the mat. Together, we will learn how to experience the joy of movement, the power of breath, and the beauty of greeting each moment with open arms. These are all things that we will learn how to do together. It is more than simply a yoga practice; it is a guide to living your life to the fullest possible extent. This is accomplished by taking one breath at a time. To begin your adventure, which is titled "28 Day Chair Yoga For Seniors," you have arrived at the beginning of your journey.

Chapter 1: Chair Yoga

When it comes to holistic wellness practices, yoga stands out as a discipline that is extremely versatile, offering a plethora of variations that may be adapted to meet a wide range of skills and requirements. Among these varieties, chair yoga stands out as an alternative that is both accessible and useful, particularly for people who are elderly or have restricted mobility. The purpose of this chapter is to delve into the fundamentals of chair yoga, including its numerous advantages for elderly citizens, as well as the essential safety considerations and precautions that are linked with its practice.

What is Chair Yoga?

One type of yoga that is considered to be mild is called chair yoga, and it is performed while sitting on a chair or utilizing a chair as a support. Through the modification of classic yoga postures, it is possible to make them accessible to persons who may have difficulties with maintaining balance, standing for extended periods of time, or getting up and down from the floor. In spite of the fact that it is conducted mostly in a seated position, chair yoga integrates components of breathwork, meditation, and moderate movement, making it an approach to wellbeing that is holistic in nature.

The versatility of chair yoga is one of the characteristics that sets it apart from other forms of yoga. In order to ensure that participants of any age, fitness level, or physical condition are able to reap the advantages of the routines, practitioners are able to tailor them to accommodate individual requirements or limits. It is also possible to practice chair yoga nearly anywhere, including in community centers, senior centers, workplaces, or even in the comfort of one's own home, which makes it an extremely convenient and accessible form of yoga.

Benefits of Chair Yoga for Seniors

In terms of both physical and mental health, senior citizens can reap a wide range of benefits from practicing chair yoga. A few of the most important benefits are as follows:

There are modest stretches and motions that are included in chair yoga, which help to improve flexibility and range of motion in the joints. This is one of the benefits of chair yoga. There are additional advantages, such as an expanded range of motion. This can be of great assistance to senior persons who may experience stiffness or restricted movement as a consequence of their disease. Age-related disorders such as osteoporosis and arthritis are examples of conditions that might be affected by this.

Participants are able to work a wide range of muscle groups while seated by performing motions and positions that are coordinated with one another. Strength and stability are both strengthened as a consequence of this. When it comes to preserving balance and lowering the risk of falling, which is a significant concern among senior citizens, strength and stability are essential components. Over time, this can result in increased strength and stability, both of which are necessary for an individual to maintain their equilibrium.

3. Stress Reduction and Relaxation: Chair yoga incorporates breathing techniques and mindfulness practices that help to reduce stress and promote relaxation. Chair yoga also helps to reduce stress. Through the practice of deep breathing exercises, one can get a sense of calmness in the nervous system, a reduction in anxiety, and an improvement in their general mental well-being.

4. Enhancements to Posture and Awareness of the Body Engaging in mindful movement and practicing optimal alignment are two ways in which senior citizens can improve their posture and achieve a greater awareness of their body. An individual can enhance their spinal health, have less discomfort in their back, and reduce the probability of being involved in an accident if they take these steps.

5. Possibilities for Social Connection and Community: Seniors who participate in chair yoga classes have the opportunity to interact with other people in an environment that is supportive and welcoming to all individuals. The development of a sense of community and social relationships can make a substantial contribution to the overall happiness and sense of well-being of an individual.

People who have limited mobility, chronic pain, or other health challenges are able to participate in the practice of chair yoga because it eliminates many of the constraints that are connected with traditional yoga practice. This makes it possible for people to be included in the practice. Through the practice of yoga while seated on a chair, the benefits of yoga can be experienced by anybody, regardless of age or physical condition. This is because yoga is a practice that can be done by anyone.

Safety Considerations and Precautions

Despite the fact that chair yoga is generally safe for older citizens, it is vital to take certain precautions in order to guarantee that the practice is both harmless and enjoyable:

1. Make an appointment with a healthcare provider. Prior to commencing any new fitness program, it is critical to communicate with your healthcare professional about your health and fitness goals. The significance of this cannot be overstated, particularly if you have any pre-existing health conditions or worries. The ability to provide tailored advice and guidance that are based on your particular needs and medical history is something that they are able to do.

2. Pay Attention to Your Physical Aspects: When you are practicing, it is essential to pay attention to how your body is feeling and to respect the restrictions that it has. To avoid overextending yourself or putting yourself into postures that are uncomfortable, it is essential to stop from doing either of these things. If you have the impression that something isn't quite right, you have the option of either switching positions or entirely ignoring it.

Ensure that you are using the appropriate technique and alignment: For the purpose of avoiding strain or injury, it is essential to pay close attention to maintaining correct alignment and technique throughout each posture. It is possible for your instructor to provide you with guidance on alignment cues and suggestions for improvements in order to guarantee that you are practicing in a secure manner.

If you want to make sure that you stay hydrated throughout your chair yoga practice, you should make sure to drink a lot of water before, during, and after your session. Additionally, this is of utmost significance if you are perspiring or pushing yourself for the entirety of your practice.

5. Remember to avoid overworking yourself: It is nevertheless possible to overexert yourself when practicing chair yoga, despite the fact that it is a low-impact and gentle type of exercise. It is especially important to keep this in mind if you are just starting out with physical activity or if you are struggling with health issues. Ensure that you keep a consistent pace and that you take rests if they are required.

6. When you need support, make use of props. Your ability to give yourself with additional support and stability can be improved by making use of props during practice. Some examples of props include blocks, blankets, and straps. The utilization of props allows for the modification of yoga poses, which not only makes them more accessible but also lessens the likelihood of becoming injured.

7. Pay Attention to the Balancing of Your Life It is recommended that you position your chair in such a way that it is close to a wall or a solid surface for support if you have difficulty keeping your balance or stability. In order to prevent

the chair from sliding, there is also the possibility of affixing rubber tips or non-slip patches to the legs of the chair.

8. Choose an Instructor Who Is Qualified with: If you are going to participate in chair yoga classes, you need to be sure that the instructor is experienced in working with older persons and is knowledgeable of how to modify postures in a way that is safe. It is recommended that you look for yoga instructors that have either specialized training or expertise in adapted yoga, or who have previous experience working with individuals who have impairments in their mobility.

Chair yoga offers older folks a multitude of benefits, including improved flexibility and strength, relaxation, and enhanced social ties. These benefits are just some of the many advantages that chair yoga offers. If older persons practice yoga in a responsible and secure manner, they will be able to reap the advantages of yoga and contribute to an overall improvement in their well-being. Chair yoga has the potential to be an advantageous addition to the wellness routine of a senior citizen, thereby boosting health and energy for many years to come. Therefore, it is important for senior citizens to take the necessary precautions and receive supervision from teachers who are knowledgeable in the field.

Chapter 2: Basic Chair Yoga Poses

In this chapter, we will explore a range of basic chair yoga poses that are accessible to practitioners of all levels. These poses are designed to promote relaxation, flexibility, and mindfulness, making them perfect for those with limited mobility or anyone looking for a gentle introduction to yoga.

1. Seated Mountain Pose:

Seated Mountain Pose, also known as Tadasana, is a foundational yoga pose that promotes good posture and alignment while cultivating a sense of strength and stability. To practice Seated Mountain Pose in a chair:

- Sit comfortably in your chair with your feet flat on the floor and your spine tall.

- Place your hands on your thighs or knees, palms facing down.

- Ground down through your sit bones and lengthen up through the crown of your head.

- Engage your abdominal muscles and relax your shoulders down away from your ears.

- Close your eyes if comfortable, and take several deep breaths, feeling rooted and grounded like a mountain.

Seated Mountain Pose is an excellent way to center yourself and bring your awareness to the present moment, preparing you for the rest of your practice.

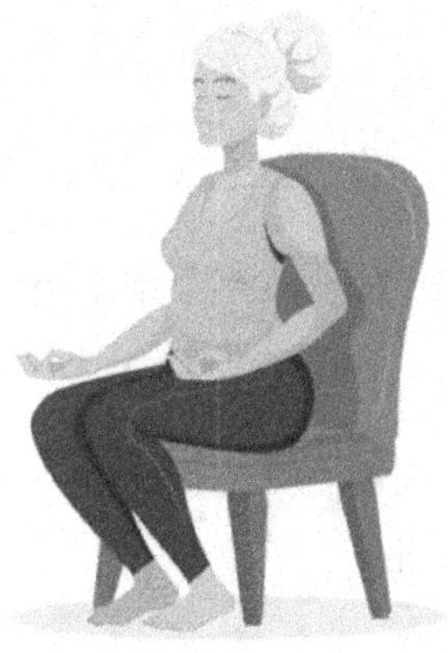

Seated Mountain Pose

Scan Video link

2. Seated Forward Bend:

Seated Forward Bend, or Paschimottanasana, stretches the entire back of the body, including the spine, hamstrings, and calves. To practice Seated Forward Bend in a chair:

- Sit near the front edge of your chair with your feet hip-width apart and flat on the floor.

- Inhale to lengthen your spine, then exhale as you hinge forward from your hips, leading with your chest.

- Allow your hands to rest on your thighs, shins, or the floor, depending on your flexibility.

- Keep your back flat and avoid rounding your spine.

- Hold the pose for several breaths, feeling a gentle stretch along the back of your body.

- To come out of the pose, inhale and slowly rise back up to a seated position.

Seated Forward Bend is a calming pose that releases tension in the back and promotes relaxation.

Seated Forward Bend

Scan Video Link:

3. Seated Twist:

Seated Twist, or Ardha Matsyendrasana, increases spinal mobility and improves digestion while also stretching the shoulders and chest. To practice Seated Twist in a chair:

- Sit up tall in your chair with your feet flat on the floor and your spine lengthened.

- Inhale to lift your arms overhead, then exhale to twist to the right, bringing your left hand to the outside of your right knee and your right hand to the back of the chair.

- Keep your spine tall as you twist, avoiding any strain or discomfort.

- Hold the twist for several breaths, gently deepening into the pose with each exhale.

- Inhale to release the twist, then repeat on the opposite side.

Seated Twist stimulates the digestive organs and helps to detoxify the body, leaving you feeling refreshed and revitalized.

Seated Twist pose, or Ardha Matsyendrasana

Scan Video Link:

4. Seated Cat-Cow Stretch:

Seated Cat-Cow Stretch combines two classic yoga poses, Cat Pose and Cow Pose, to promote spinal flexibility and mobility. To practice Seated Cat-Cow Stretch in a chair:

- Sit comfortably in your chair with your feet flat on the floor and your hands resting on your thighs.

- Inhale to arch your back and lift your chest, drawing your shoulder blades together (Cow Pose).

- Exhale to round your spine, tucking your chin to your chest and drawing your belly button toward your spine (Cat Pose).

- Continue flowing between Cat and Cow Poses with your breath, moving smoothly and mindfully.

- Focus on synchronizing your movement with your breath, allowing each inhale to lift and open your heart, and each exhale to round and release your spine.

Seated Cat-Cow Stretch is a gentle warm-up for the spine, perfect for relieving tension and improving posture.

Seated Cat-Cow Stretch pose

Scan Video Link:

5. Seated Side Stretch:

Seated Side Stretch targets the muscles along the sides of the body, including the intercostal muscles and obliques, while also stretching the arms and shoulders. To practice Seated Side Stretch in a chair:

- Sit comfortably in your chair with your feet flat on the floor and your spine tall.

- Inhale to lengthen your spine, then exhale as you reach your right arm up and over to the left, stretching through the right side of your body.

- Keep both sit bones grounded on the chair and avoid collapsing into the stretch.

- Hold the stretch for several breaths, feeling a deep opening along the right side of your body.

- Inhale to come back to center, then exhale and repeat on the opposite side.

Seated Side Stretch is a rejuvenating pose that increases lateral mobility and expands the breath.

Seated Side Stretch

Scan Video Link:

6. **Seated Sun Salutation:**

Seated Sun Salutation offers a modified version of the traditional Sun Salutation sequence, providing a full-body stretch and energizing flow from the comfort of a chair. To practice Seated Sun Salutation:

- Sit near the front edge of your chair with your feet hip-width apart and flat on the floor.

- Inhale to reach your arms overhead, lengthening through your fingertips.

- Exhale to hinge forward from your hips, bringing your chest toward your thighs in Seated Forward Bend.

- Inhale to lift halfway up, lengthening your spine and reaching your heart forward.

- Exhale to fold forward again, releasing any tension in the neck and shoulders.

- Inhale to rise all the way up to seated, sweeping your arms out to the sides and up overhead.

- Exhale to bring your hands to heart center, grounding down through your sit bones and centering your energy.

When performed in a seated position, the Sun Salutation sequence is a dynamic routine that improves flexibility, increases circulation, and enhances general well-being.

Seated Sun Salutation

Scan Video Link:

If you implement these fundamental chair yoga positions into your daily practice, you may find that you have a greater sense of equilibrium, flexibility, and centering in both your body and your mind. Take your time with each pose, paying attention to what your body is telling you, and making adjustments as necessary to discover the one that feels most comfortable for you. It is possible that as you continue to practice yoga, you will discover that certain postures become easier to do. This will enable you to participate in the full advantages of yoga without having to leave the comfort of your chair.

Building Strength and Flexibility

Chair yoga can be an effective approach to increase strength and flexibility, in addition to fostering relaxation and mindfulness. Chair yoga exercises can be performed in a chair. In this section, we will investigate three chair yoga postures that have been developed with the specific intention of enhancing flexibility in the legs and hips as well as strengthening the core muscles.

1. **Seated Abdominal Twists:**

The abdominal muscles, obliques, and lower back are all targeted by the seated abdominal twists, which are also known as the Bharadvajasana Twist. Additionally, the spinal mobility is improved by performing these twists. When performing seated abdominal twists, you should:

- Assume a tall seated position in your chair, with your feet planted firmly on the ground and your spine stretched out.

- To provide yourself with support, position your hands on the armrests or the back of the chair.

- Take a deep breath in to stretch your spine, and then exhale to twist to the right. As you do this, bring your left hand to the outside of your right leg, and bring your right hand behind you on the chair where you are sitting.

- To prevent collapsing into the twist, it is important to keep both sit bones firmly planted on the chair.

- If you feel comfortable doing so, look over your right shoulder while strengthening the twist with each exhalation.

- The twist should be held for many breaths, and you should feel a slight compression in the abdominal region.

- To return to the center, take a deep breath in, then exhale and repeat the process on the opposite side.

Seated Abdominal Twists strengthen the core muscles and promote detoxification by massaging the internal organs.

Seated Abdominal Twists

Scan Video Link:

2. Seated Leg Lifts:

Seated Leg Lifts target the quadriceps, hip flexors, and abdominal muscles, helping to build strength and stability in the lower body. To practice Seated Leg Lifts:

- You should position yourself so that your feet are flat on the floor and your hands are resting on your thighs. Sit close to the front edge of your chair.

- When you inhale, your spine will lengthen, and you will engage your abdominal muscles to provide support.

- You should exhale in order to extend your right leg forward and lift it off the floor while maintaining a flexed foot position.

- Make sure that your knee is straight and that your spine is tall while you hold the leg lift for a few breaths.

- After bringing your right foot back down to the floor with an inhalation, exhale and repeat the exercise with your left foot.

- For a number of repetitions, continue to alternate between lifting your right leg and your left leg, making sure to keep your control and stability throughout the entire exercise.

Seated Leg Lifts improve balance, strengthen the muscles of the legs, and enhance overall lower body function.

Seated Leg Lifts

Scan Video Link:

3. **Seated Boat Pose Variation:**

Seated Boat Pose Variation is a modified version of the classic Boat Pose (Navasana), which strengthens the core muscles and improves balance and stability. To practice Seated Boat Pose Variation:

- Position yourself so that your feet are planted firmly on the ground and your hands are resting on the armrests or the sides of the chair. Sit close to the front edge of your chair chair.

- By inhaling, you can stretch your spine and engage the muscles in your abdominal region.

- When you exhale, you should lean back slightly, lift your feet off the floor, and bring your knees closer to your chest since you are doing this.

- Maintain a tall posture by holding onto the edges of the chair for support. Keep your chest high and your spine lifted.

- Extend your arms forward side by side with your legs, parallel to the ground, if you feel comfortable doing so.

- Continue to hold the pose for a few breaths while you feel the muscles in your core muscles contracting.

- Release the position by taking a deep breath in and bringing your feet back down to the floor in a controlled manner.

The abdominal muscles are strengthened, posture is improved, and core stability and balance are enhanced with the use of the Seated Boat Pose Variation workout.

Seated Boat Pose Variation

Scan Video Link:

Your practice of chair yoga can help you grow a stronger, more resilient body while also boosting general well-being if you incorporate these postures that build strength and enhance flexibility into your routine. It is crucial to pay attention to your body, move thoughtfully, and respect your limitations whether you are participating in any kind of fitness program. You will progressively acquire strength, flexibility, and confidence in your chair yoga practice if you practice it on a regular basis and have patience.

Enhancing Balance and Stability

When it comes to our physical well-being, balance and stability are quite important, particularly as we become older. Balance and stability can be improved via the practice of chair yoga, which also helps to increase focus and concentration. Chair yoga is a gentle yet effective method. Within the scope of this part, we will investigate three chair yoga postures that have been specifically intended to improve balanced and stable posture.

1. Chair Warrior Pose:

Chair Warrior Pose is a modified version of the traditional Warrior Pose (Virabhadrasana), which strengthens the legs, opens the hips, and improves balance and concentration. To practice Chair Warrior Pose:

- Position yourself so that your feet are flat on the floor and your spine is tall. Sit close to the front edge of your chair.

- Put your right foot in a flexed position and extend your right leg straight out in front of you. Make sure that your toes are pointed upward.

- Position your left foot so that it is firmly planted on the floor behind you, with your toes facing slightly outward. Step your left foot back behind you.

- To reach your arms overhead, take a deep breath in and maintain a comfortable posture with your shoulders and your gaze forward.

- While maintaining a straight and powerful back leg, exhale to sink into your front knee and bend it to a 90-degree angle. Additionally, keep your rear leg straight.

- As you hold the pose for a number of breaths, you should feel a sense of solidity and grounding through your legs and core.

- As you come back up to standing, take a deep breath in, then exhale and repeat the process on the other side.

Chair Warrior Pose strengthens the legs, improves balance, and cultivates mental focus and determination.

Chair Warrior Pose

Scan Video Link

2. Chair Tree Pose:

Chair Tree Pose is a modified version of the classic Tree Pose (Vrksasana), which improves balance, stability, and concentration while also stretching the hips and inner thighs. To practice Chair Tree Pose:

- Sit near the front edge of your chair with your feet flat on the floor and your spine tall.

- Shift your weight into your left foot, rooting down through the four corners of the foot.

- Lift your right foot off the floor and place the sole of your right foot on the inside of your left calf or thigh, avoiding the knee joint.

- Press your foot into your leg and your leg into your foot, finding stability and support.

- Inhale to reach your arms overhead, bringing your palms together in prayer position or extending your fingertips toward the ceiling.

- Engage your core muscles and find a focal point to help you maintain balance.

- Hold the pose for several breaths, feeling rooted and stable like a tree in the wind.

- Inhale to release the pose, lowering your right foot back to the floor, and repeat on the opposite side.

Chair Tree Pose improves balance, strengthens the muscles of the legs and core, and enhances concentration and focus.

Chair Tree Pose senior

Scan Video Link:

3. Chair Dancer Pose:

Chair Dancer Pose is a modified version of the classic Dancer Pose (Natarajasana), which improves balance, flexibility, and strength while also opening the chest and shoulders. To practice Chair Dancer Pose:

- Position yourself so that your feet are flat on the floor and your spine is tall. Sit close to the front edge of your chair.

- Make sure that your weight is shifting into your left foot, and then extend your right leg in front of you in a straight line.

- Put your right hand behind your back and grab the inside of your right foot or ankle while keeping your knees close together. This will help you with the exercise.

- Exhale to hinge forward from your hips, thrusting your right foot into your hand and rising your chest. Inhale to extend your spine, and then exhale to hinge forward from within your hips.

- In order to achieve equilibrium and stability, extend your left arm forward until it is at shoulder height.

- During the time that you hold the pose for a number of breaths, you should feel a profound stretch in the front of your body as well as an opening in your heart.

- Release the pose by taking a deep breath in and bringing your right foot back down to the floor. Repeat the process on the other side of your body.

Chair Dancer Pose improves balance, flexibility, and strength while also promoting openness and expansiveness in both body and mind.

Chair Dancer Pose:

Scan Video Link:

Integration and Beyond

Through the practice of seated sun salutation and a chair yoga flow sequence, we will investigate the integration of breath with movement in this section of the article. During your practice, these sequences are intended to assist you in establishing a connection between your mind, body, and breath, thereby fostering a sense of flow, balance, and vigor.

1. Seated Sun Salutation:

Seated Sun Salutation is a modified variation of the conventional Sun Salutation sequence. It provides a soothing flow of movements that stimulate the body and boost the spirit during the practice. Both as a stand-alone routine and as a warm-up for additional chair yoga postures, this sequence can be practiced in either orientation.

Posture yourself so that you are sat in a comfortable position toward the front edge of your chair. Place both of your feet firmly on the floor, and make sure that your spine is tall. Allow yourself some time to center yourself and get more in tune with your breath.

a. Mountain Pose (Tadasana):

- Inhale as you reach your arms overhead, lengthening through your fingertips.

- Exhale as you bring your palms together in prayer position at your heart center, grounding down through your sit bones.

b. Seated Forward Bend (Uttanasana):

- Inhale to lengthen your spine, then exhale as you hinge forward from your hips, leading with your chest.

- Allow your hands to rest on your thighs, shins, or the floor, depending on your flexibility.

- Hold the forward bend for a few breaths, feeling a gentle stretch along the back of your body.

c. Seated Halfway Lift (Ardha Uttanasana):

- Inhale to lift halfway up, lengthening your spine and reaching your heart forward.

- Keep your back flat and your chest open, engaging your abdominal muscles for support.

d. Seated Forward Bend (Uttanasana):

- Exhale to fold forward again, releasing any tension in the neck and shoulders.

- Allow your head to hang heavy, surrendering to the stretch in your spine and hamstrings.

e. Mountain Pose (Tadasana):

- Inhale to rise all the way up to seated, sweeping your arms out to the sides and up overhead.

- Reach up towards the sky, lengthening through your fingertips and lifting your heart.

f. Hands to Heart Center:

- Exhale as you bring your hands back to heart center, grounding down through your sit bones and centering your energy.

- Take a moment to pause and reconnect with your breath before moving on to the next pose or sequence.

When performed in a seated position, the Sun Salutation sequence is a dynamic routine that improves flexibility, increases circulation, and enhances general well-being. When you practice, make sure you do so with conscious awareness, moving in tune with your breath, and paying attention to the requirements of your body.

2. Chair Yoga Flow Sequence:

Strength, flexibility, balance, and mindfulness are all enhanced by the Chair Yoga Flow Sequence, which is a dynamic series of poses that flow together in a seamless manner. It is possible to modify this sequence in order to cater to your specific requirements and preferences, which makes it suitable for practitioners of various professional levels.

Posture yourself so that you are sat in a comfortable position toward the front edge of your chair. Place both of your feet firmly on the floor, and make sure that your spine is tall. Spend some time bringing your attention inward and establishing a connection with your breath.

a. Seated Mountain Pose:

- Inhale as you reach your arms overhead, lengthening through your fingertips.

- Exhale as you bring your palms together in prayer position at your heart center, grounding down through your sit bones.

b. Seated Twist:

- Inhale to lengthen your spine, then exhale as you twist to the right, bringing your left hand to the outside of your right knee and your right hand to the back of the chair.

- Keep your spine tall and your chest open, gazing over your right shoulder if comfortable.

c. Seated Side Stretch:

- Inhale to return to center, then exhale as you reach your right arm up and over to the left, stretching through the right side of your body.

- Keep both sit bones grounded on the chair and avoid collapsing into the stretch.

d. Seated Cat-Cow Stretch:

- Inhale to arch your back and lift your chest (Cow Pose), then exhale to round your spine and tuck your chin to your chest (Cat Pose).

- Flow between Cat and Cow Poses with your breath, moving mindfully and fluidly.

e. Seated Forward Bend:

- Inhale to lengthen your spine, then exhale as you hinge forward from your hips, leading with your chest.

- Allow your hands to rest on your thighs, shins, or the floor, finding a position that feels comfortable and supportive.

f. Seated Warrior Pose:

- Inhale to sweep your arms out to the sides and up overhead, reaching up towards the sky.

- Exhale as you bring your palms together in prayer position at your heart center, grounding down through your sit bones.

g. Seated Tree Pose:

- Inhale to extend your right leg out to the side, placing the sole of your right foot on the inner thigh or calf of your left leg.

- Exhale as you bring your hands back to heart center, finding balance and stability in the pose.

h. Seated Dancer Pose:

- Inhale to reach your right arm up towards the sky, then exhale as you lean to the left, extending your right leg out to the side and reaching your right hand towards your left foot.

- Find a gentle stretch along the right side of your body, keeping your spine tall and your chest open.

i. Return to Center:

- Inhale to return to center, bringing your hands back to heart center and your right foot back to the floor.

- Take a moment to pause and reconnect with your breath before moving on to the next side or pose.

Strength, flexibility, balance, and awareness are all enhanced through the practice of the Chair Yoga Flow Sequence, which is a dynamic and stimulating exercise routine. Move gracefully and with focus, allowing your breath to lead you through each stance and transition as you move through the poses. Through consistent practice, you will be able to create a more profound sense of connection and well-being in both your spirit and your body.

Chapter 3: Breathing Techniques

A person's ability to breathe is one of the most essential functions of their body. On the other hand, it is frequently disregarded when it comes to the management of stress, the enhancement of focus, and the general improvement of well-being. The purpose of this chapter is to look into a variety of breathing practices that have been performed for centuries across a wide range of nations and traditions. Relaxation, clarity, and inner peace are all promoted via the use of these techniques, which give tremendous advantages for both the mind and the body. This lesson will focus on four important breathing exercises: breathing with the diaphragm, breathing with the alternate nostril, breathing with the ujjayi, and counting breaths.

Diaphragmatic Breathing

One kind of breathing that requires the use of the diaphragm, which is a big muscle positioned at the base of the lungs, is called diaphragmatic breathing. This method is also referred to as belly breathing or abdominal breathing. It is normal for infants to breathe in this manner, but as we get older, this type of breathing tends to decrease and is frequently replaced with chest breathing that is shallower. Due to the fact that it is easy to learn and can be done anywhere, diaphragmatic breathing is an efficient method for lowering tension and increasing relaxation.

How to Practice Diaphragmatic Breathing:

1. Determine a Position That Is Comfortable: Sit or lie down in a position that is comfortable for you. If you would choose, you are free to close your eyes.

2. Put your hand on your stomach and look down. Place one hand on your stomach, down below your rib cage, and hold it there. The other hand should be placed on your chest.

3. Inhale Slowly: Take a slow breath in through your nose, allowing your stomach to rise as you do so. It is important to concentrate on moving your hand out with your breath while maintaining a somewhat still chest motion.

4. Exhale Slowly: Exhale via your mouth or nose, allowing your abdomen to sag as you let the breath out of your body.

5. Repeat: Carry on with this pattern of breathing for a few minutes, concentrating on the feeling of your abdominal region rising and falling with each breath.

Benefits of Diaphragmatic Breathing:

- The relaxation response in the body is activated by diaphragmatic breathing, which results in a reduction in the levels of stress hormones such as cortisol and a promotion of a sense of tranquility.

- Increased Oxygenation: When you fully engage the diaphragm, you increase the amount of oxygen that enters your lungs. This increased oxygenation can improve the overall oxygenation of the body as well as the levels of energy that are available.

- Enhanced Digestion: The vagus nerve, which is responsible for digestion and relaxation, is stimulated by deep breathing, which results in enhanced digestion. When it comes to digestive disorders like bloating and indigestion, practicing diaphragmatic breathing may be helpful in alleviating these symptoms.

- Lower Blood Pressure: According to research, practicing diaphragmatic breathing on a regular basis can help lower blood pressure levels, which in turn reduces the chance of developing hypertension and cardiovascular disease.

- Increased Mindfulness: You can cultivate mindfulness and present-moment awareness by concentrating on the sensations of your breathing. This can help you improve your ability to concentrate and your mental clarity.

How to Practice Diaphragmatic Breathing:

Scan Video Link:

Alternate Nostril Breathing

A yogic breathing practice known as alternate nostril breathing is designed to bring about a state of equilibrium in the flow of energy throughout the body. Alternating the breath between the left and right nostrils is a technique that is claimed to generate a sense of equilibrium and bring about harmony between the two hemispheres of the brain.

How to Practice Alternate Nostril Breathing:

1. Ensure that you are seated in a comfortable position and that your spine is in an upright position. You have the option of sitting on the floor with your legs crossed or sitting on a chair, whatever is more comfortable for you.

2. Get ready to take a big breath: The palm of your left hand should be facing upward as you place it on your left knee. Position your right hand so that it is facing your face.

3. **Make Use Of Your Right Thumb:** Make use of your right thumb to pull your right nostril closed, and then take a deep breath in through your left nostril.

4. **Reverse the Sides:** Your right ring finger should be used to close your left nostril while you let go of your right nose. Finish your exhalation by exhaling through your right nostril.

5. **Inhale Through Right Nostril** While keeping your left nose closed, take a deep breath in through your right nostril.

6. **Flip the Switch Once More:** Your left nostril should be released, and your right thumb should be used to shut your right nose. Make sure that you exhale completely via your left nostril.

7. **Repetition of the Cycle:** Carry on with this alternating pattern for a number of rounds, making sure that each inhale and exhale is slow, steady, and under control.

Benefits of Alternate Nostril Breathing:

- Energy Channels Are Balanced: According to yogic philosophy, the left nostril is related with the lunar energy known as ida, which is a relaxing energy, while the right nostril is associated with the solar energy known as pingala, which is an invigorating energy. Maintaining a sense of harmony and equilibrium can be accomplished by alternating between the two nostrils, which will allow you to bring these energy pathways into balance.

- Bringing to a state of profound relaxation, the rhythmic pattern of alternate nostril breathing can bring about a sense of calmness in the mind, hence reducing emotions of anxiety and stress.

- Improves Cognitive Function and Enhances Mental Clarity It is claimed that this breathing method can improve cognitive function and enhance mental clarity by coordinating the activity of the left and right hemispheres of the brain.

- Supports Respiratory Health: Alternate nostril breathing can assist in clearing the nasal passages and improving respiratory function. As a result, it is good for persons who suffer from allergies, sinus congestion, or respiratory problems.

- Through the regulation of the flow of prana, also known as life force energy, in the body, alternate nostril breathing can assist in the regulation of emotions and the promotion of emotional stability.

How to Practice Alternate Nostril Breathing

Scan Video Link:

Ujjayi Breath

One of the pranayama (breathing) techniques that is frequently utilized in yoga practice is the ujjayi breath, which is also referred to as the ocean breath or the victorious breath. When performing this technique of deep, audible breathing, the back of the neck is somewhat constricted, which results in the production of a faint whispering sound that is reminiscent of ocean waves. Yoga postures, also known as asanas, are frequently combined with the practice of ujjayi breath in order to improve focus, generate heat within the body, and cultivate mindfulness.

How to Practice Ujjayi Breath:

1. Put yourself in a comfortable position by sitting or lying down in a position that is pleasant for you. Make sure that your spine is straight and that your shoulders are relaxed.

2. Slowly inhale via your nose: Take a deep breath in through your nose, allowing your lungs to be filled with air. Create a soft hissing or whispering sound by slightly contracting the muscles at the back of your throat when you inhale. This will help you speak more clearly.

3. Exhale Slowly Through Your Nose: In order to produce the same whispering sound, you should exhale slowly

and steadily through your nose while keeping a tiny tightness in your throat.

4. Pay Attention to the Sound: As your breath enters and exits your body, pay attention to the sound that it makes. Imagine you are listening to a sound that is similar to the ebb and flow of waves in the ocean.

5. Maintain a Consistent Rhythm: If you are performing yoga asanas, continue this rhythmic breathing pattern, making sure to synchronize your breath with your movements.

Benefits of Ujjayi Breath:

- Enhances Mindfulness: The audible character of Ujjayi breath acts as a focal point for mindfulness, assisting in the anchoring of your consciousness in the present now and helping to calm the chattering of the mind.

- Ujjayi breath is a good technique for warming up the muscles and enhancing flexibility during yoga practice since it generates heat within the body. This makes it an excellent technique for yoga practice.

- Increases Concentration: Ujjayi breath helps sharpen concentration and deepen meditative states by integrating breath with movement and retaining awareness of the sound of the breath. This helps achieve the goal of improving concentration.

- Controls the Flow of Energy The rhythmic quality of the Ujjayi breath controls the flow of prana, which is the energy that is associated with life force, throughout the body, which in turn promotes balance and vigor.

- Relaxes and Calms the Nervous System The slow and constant pattern of Ujjayi breath stimulates the parasympathetic nervous system, which results in a feeling of relaxation and tranquility.

How to Practice Ujjayi Breath:

Scan Video Link:

Breath Counting

Breath counting is a mindfulness technique that involves counting the breaths as a means of anchoring attention and developing mental clarity. For example, you could count the number of breaths you take. The mind may be trained to remain focused and present via the use of this straightforward yet effective technique, which makes it a useful instrument for the management of stress and the improvement of overall well-being.

How to Practice Breath Counting:

1. **Find a Calm Place:** Sit in a comfortable position in a place where you won't be bothered and where there is a somewhat quiet atmosphere.

2. To relax both your body and your mind, close your eyes gently and take a few deep breaths. This will help you relax thoroughly.

3. **Start Counting:** While you are taking a breath in, mentally count "one" via your nose. Count "two" as you let out your breath. Maintain the counting of each inhale and exhale until you reach a predetermined number, such as five or 10 consecutive counts.

4. **Begin Again:** When you have reached the number you have set for yourself, begin again from the beginning. If you discover that you have lost track of the number or that your mind has wandered, return your focus back to the breath in a gentle manner and start counting again from one.

5. **Practice on a regular basis:** Your goal should be to practice counting breaths for a few minutes every day, and as you become more familiar with the technique, you should gradually increase the duration of your practice.

Benefits of Breath Counting:

- When you count your breaths, you train your mind to remain focused on the here and now, which improves your ability to concentrate and maintain attentional control.

- The practice of counting breaths helps to calm the mind by focusing attention on the breath itself. This helps to quiet the mind's constant chatter, which in turn promotes a sense of inner peace and calmness.

- Increases Self-Awareness: Counting breaths is a practice that helps enhance self-awareness by bringing attention to the breath and the subtle sensations that are connected with breathing.

- As a result of the rhythmic pattern of counting breaths, the body's relaxation response is activated, which in turn reduces stress levels and promotes emotional well-being.

- Enhances Mental Clarity: Counting breaths on a regular basis can help improve mental clarity and cognitive function, making it simpler to make decisions and find solutions to issues.

How to Practice Breath Counting:

Scan Video Link:

Breathing techniques offer powerful tools for promoting relax, alleviate stress, and improve overall well-being are all goals of relaxing. It doesn't matter if you want to enhance your physical health, develop your mindfulness, or relax your mind; there is a breathing technique that will help you achieve all of these goals. Through persistent practice, these techniques can be simply incorporated into daily life. From the straightforwardness of diaphragmatic breathing to the complexities of alternate nostril breathing and ujjayi breath, these techniques can be effortlessly incorporated. You are able to create a deeper connection to yourself and the present moment by harnessing the power of the breath, which will ultimately lead to increased clarity, tranquility, and vitality in all parts of your life. Now is the time to take a few deep breaths and go on the journey to achieving inner balance and well-being.

Chapter 4: Daily Yoga Routine

It might be difficult to find the time to devote to a thorough yoga practice in the modern world, which moves at a breakneck pace. On the other hand, including chair yoga into your daily routine can provide a multitude of advantages, such as increased flexibility, improved posture, decreased stress, and an overall improvement in well-being. The Morning Chair Yoga Sequence, the Afternoon Chair Yoga Sequence, and the Evening Chair Yoga Sequence are the three chair yoga sequences that we will introduce in this chapter. Each of these sequences is meant to be easily incorporated into your daily routine. It is possible to practice these sequences in the convenience of your own home or office, and they are appropriate for people of all ages and levels of fitness.

Morning Chair Yoga Sequence

With this invigorating Morning Chair Yoga Sequence, you can get your day off to a productive and revitalizing start. The purpose of this sequence is to prepare you for the day ahead by having you awaken both your body and your mind via the use of focused breathing and mild stretches.

1. Seated Cat-Cow Stretch:

    - Position yourself in a comfortable chair with your feet planted firmly on the ground and hip-width apart.

    - Your hands should be placed on your knees.

- By arching your back and elevating your chest while tilting your pelvis forward, you should take a deep breath in (Cow Pose).

- Relax your spine and exhale as you bring your chin to your chest and round your spine (Cat Pose).

- Continue this flowing movement for five to ten breaths, making sure to synchronize your breathing with your movement.

2. Seated Side Stretch:

- Remain erect in your chair and place both feet firmly on the ground.

- Take a deep breath in and raise your right arm above your head, extending it toward the ceiling.

- When you feel a stretch down the right side of your body, exhale and lean gently to the left with your left hand.

- Observe for three to five breaths, and then switch sides.

3. Seated Forward Fold:

- Take a seat with your feet hip-width apart and your back to the front edge of the chair.

- Taking a deep breath, stretch your spine.

- As you exhale, tilt forward from your hips and reach your hands toward your feet or the floor until you reach your hands.

- For three to five breaths, hold this position until you feel a stretch along the back of your legs and spine.

4. Seated Spinal Twist:

- Remain erect in your chair and place both feet firmly on the ground.

- Taking a deep breath, stretch your spine.

- As you exhale, twist to the right while placing your left hand on your right knee and your right hand on the back of the chair. After this, repeat the exercise.

- First, hold for three to five breaths, and then repeat on the other side.

5. Seated Sun Salutation:

- Keep your feet planted firmly on the ground and sit properly on your chair.

- Make sure your palms are facing each other as you inhale and stretch your arms upward (Mountain Pose).

- As you exhale, bring your hands together in front of your heart and keep them there (Prayer Position).

- Perform this routine three to five times while being in sync with your breathing.

Afternoon Chair Yoga Sequence

The calming Afternoon Chair Yoga Sequence is a great way to combat exhaustion during the middle of the day and to revitalize both your body and your mind. By releasing stress and increasing your energy levels via the use of these easy stretches and mindful exercises, you will be able to end the day in a strong and confident manner.

1. Seated Neck Stretch:

    - Sit tall in your chair, feet flat on the floor.

    - Inhale and lengthen your spine.

    - Exhale and drop your right ear towards your right shoulder, feeling a stretch along the left side of your neck.

    - Hold for 3-5 breaths, then switch sides.

2. Seated Shoulder Rolls:

    - Sit comfortably on your chair, feet flat on the floor.

    - Inhale as you lift your shoulders towards your ears.

    - Exhale and roll your shoulders back and down.

- Repeat this movement for 5-10 breaths, then reverse the direction.

3. Seated Side Bend:

   - Sit tall in your chair, feet flat on the floor.

   - Inhale and reach your arms overhead, clasping your hands together.

   - Exhale and lean gently to the right, feeling a stretch along the left side of your body.

   - Hold for 3-5 breaths, then switch sides.

4. Seated Pigeon Pose:

   - Sit towards the front edge of your chair, feet hip-width apart.

   - Cross your right ankle over your left knee, flexing your right foot.

   - Inhale and lengthen your spine.

   - Exhale and hinge forward from your hips, keeping your back flat.

   - Hold for 3-5 breaths, then switch sides.

5. Seated Heart Opener:

   - Sit tall in your chair, feet flat on the floor.

   - Interlace your fingers behind your back, squeezing your shoulder blades together.

- Inhale as you lift your chest towards the ceiling, opening your heart.

- Hold for 3-5 breaths, then release.

Evening Chair Yoga Sequence

By doing this relaxing Evening Chair Yoga Sequence, you may help yourself wind down and get ready for a pleasant night's sleep. A sensation of inner calm and profound relaxation can be achieved by the practice of these easy stretches and relaxation exercises, which will assist in the release of tension that has built up throughout the day.

1. Seated Child's Pose:

    - Sit comfortably on your chair, feet flat on the floor.

    - Inhale and lengthen your spine.

    - Exhale and fold forward, resting your chest on your thighs and your forehead on your crossed arms.

    - Hold for 5-10 breaths, allowing your breath to deepen with each exhale.

2. Seated Forward Bend with Legs Extended:

    - Sit towards the front edge of your chair, legs extended straight in front of you.

    - Inhale and lengthen your spine.

- Exhale and hinge forward from your hips, reaching your hands towards your feet or the floor.

- Hold for 5-10 breaths, surrendering to the stretch with each exhale.

3. Seated Eagle Arms:

   - Sit tall in your chair, feet flat on the floor.

   - Inhale and stretch your arms out to the sides at shoulder height.

   - Exhale and cross your right arm over your left, wrapping your forearms and bringing your palms together (or holding onto opposite shoulders).

   - Hold for 3-5 breaths, then switch sides.

4. Seated Twisting Forward Fold:

   - Sit towards the front edge of your chair, feet hip-width apart.

   - Inhale and lengthen your spine.

   - Exhale and twist to the right, placing your left hand on your right knee and your right hand on the back of the chair.

   - Inhale to lengthen your spine again.

- Exhale and hinge forward from your hips, reaching your hands towards your feet or the floor.

- Hold for 3-5 breaths, feeling a gentle twist and stretch along your spine and side body.

- Repeat on the opposite side.

5. Seated Relaxation Meditation:

- Sit comfortably on your chair, feet flat on the floor.

- Close your eyes and bring your attention to your breath.

- Take slow, deep breaths, allowing each exhale to release tension from your body and mind.

- Stay in this relaxed state for 5-10 minutes, focusing on the sensation of peace and tranquility within.

Chapter 5: Balance and Stability

Enhancing Physical Wellness

When it comes to achieving the highest possible level of physical fitness, balance and stability serve as the foundational pillars that support every movement and activity that we engage in. When it comes to our general health and functionality, our capacity to maintain equilibrium and stability is essential. This is true whether we are engaging in the straightforward activity of walking or the more involved activity of lifting weights. In Chapter 5, we delve into the fundamental components of balance and stability, providing insights into chair yoga postures for the purpose of improving balance, exercises that focus on proprioception, and strategies that strengthen the core. Individuals have the capacity to build better balance and stability by taking a holistic approach that encompasses the mind, body, and spirit. This can result in an improvement in their quality of life and overall well-being.

Chair Yoga Poses for Balance Improvement

The practice of yoga, which has its origins in India and dates back to ancient times, has gained international attention for the overall advantages it offers, which include improvements in physical, mental, and emotional health. Chair yoga is a more accessible alternative to conventional yoga, particularly for individuals who have mobility constraints or physical issues. Traditional yoga typically entails elaborate poses and sequences that are performed on a mat while chair yoga offers a more straightforward approach. Because it places an emphasis on gentle movements, breathwork, and mindfulness practices, chair yoga is suited for people of all ages and fitness levels from beginners to advanced practitioners.

Within the field of improving one's balance, chair yoga provides a plethora of useful poses that are aimed at strengthening major muscle groups and improving overall stability. These postures, which are performed with the use of a strong chair for support, make it possible to make progressive progress toward improved balance and coordination. Several popular chair yoga positions that are known to improve balance include the following:

1. Individuals sit tall in a chair, anchoring their feet into the floor, engaging their core, and elongating their spine in order to achieve the exercise known as Tadasana, which is also known as Seated Mountain Pose. Through the cultivation of alignment, awareness of posture, and stability, this position lays the groundwork for enhanced balance throughout the body.

2. When performing the chair cat-cow stretch, individuals conduct moderate spinal movements by arching and rounding their backs, similar to the motions of a cat and cow. This stretch is performed while the individual is seated at the edge of a chair. Enhancing spine flexibility, fostering proprioception, and supporting general balance are all benefits that come from this fluid motion.

3. While seated in a sideways position on a chair, individuals perform the seated twist, also known as Ardha Matsyendrasana. This pose involves gradually twisting the torso while stretching one hand behind the chair and the other hand to the knee of the opposite side. Through the use of controlled rotational motions, this pose promotes spinal mobility, improves digestion, and helps cultivate equilibrium.

4. With one hand resting on the back of a chair for support, persons elevate one foot and place it on the opposite inner thigh or calf. They do this while maintaining their balance and concentrating on a fixed point in front of them. This pose is known as Chair Tree Pose (Vrksasana). In addition to improving concentration and stability, this variant of the conventional tree posture helps strengthen the leg that is at the standing position.

5. During the seated forward bend, also known as Paschimottanasana, individuals hinge at the hips and fold forward, stretching their arms towards their feet or shins. This position is performed when the individual is seated at the front edge of a chair with their feet hip-width apart. The hamstrings, calves, and lower back are all stretched out during this seated forward bend, which helps to improve flexibility and awareness of posture position.

Individuals have the opportunity to progressively improve their sense of well-being, as well as their balance and stability, by including these chair yoga poses into their everyday practice. Additionally, the use of mindful breathing techniques contributes to the promotion of relaxation, the reduction of stress, and mental clarity, which complements the physical benefits of the practice.

Proprioception Exercises
Nurturing Body Awareness

The term "proprioception," which is frequently referred to as the "sixth sense" of the body, describes the internal capacity of the body to perceive its position, movement, and orientation in space. This sensory feedback system is extremely important in ensuring that we are able to retain our equilibrium, coordination, and spatial awareness, which in turn enables us to traverse the world with precision and self-assurance. Through the use of specific motions and sensory stimulation, proprioception exercises are aimed to heighten this sense, so sharpening our bodily awareness and strengthening our stability.

The single-leg stance is a useful exercise for improving proprioception. In this exercise, individuals stand on one leg while maintaining their balance and stability. It is possible for individuals to gradually improve their proprioceptive feedback and develop their stabilizing muscles by gradually increasing the duration of this stance and introducing obstacles such as closing their eyes or standing on an unstable surface.

An additional beneficial form of exercise is the heel-to-toe walk, which is also referred to as the tandem walk. For the purpose of this exercise, participants walk in a straight line, bringing the heel of one foot directly in front of the toes of the opposing foot with each step they take. This purposeful movement pattern necessitates precise coordination and proprioceptive input, which ultimately results in enhanced balance and understanding of spatial relationships.

It is also possible to incorporate wobble cushions or balancing boards into workouts in order to provide dynamic proprioceptive input. This feedback challenges the body to maintain equilibrium and react to slight alterations in weight distribution. Due to the fact that these tools imitate real-life circumstances in which balance and coordination are regularly challenged, they provide great chances for proprioceptive training and growth.

By performing proprioception exercises on a regular basis, individuals are able to fine-tune the sensory feedback mechanisms in their bodies, which ultimately leads to improved stability, coordination, and overall physical confidence. Athletes who are looking to improve their performance can benefit from these exercises, but individuals who are trying to navigate their daily routines with better ease and precision can also profit from them.

Core Strengthening Techniques
Building Stability from Within

As the body's powerhouse, the core muscles, which include the abdominals, obliques, lower back, and pelvic floor muscles, are responsible for providing stability, support, and protection for the spine and the tissues that surround it. It is crucial to strengthen these muscles not just for the purpose of improving posture and lowering the risk of injury, but also for the purpose of significantly increasing general balance and stability. Strength, endurance, and functional stability can be better developed through the utilization of a variety of techniques and exercises that specifically target the core muscles.

1. Variations on the Plank: Planks are well-known for their effectiveness in strengthening the complete collection of muscles that make up the core. In the conventional plank posture, the arms are held in a straight line, and the body is arranged in a straight line from the head to the heels. In order to target different muscle groups inside the core, variations of planks, such as side planks, forearm planks, and planks with leg lifts, give a variety of challenges and make the exercise more challenging.

2. This exercise focuses on the oblique muscles, which are essential for rotational motions and lateral stability. The Russian Twist is a key exercise for targeting these muscles. Individuals twist their body from side to side while seated on the floor with their knees bent and their feet lifted. This exercise engages the obliques and promotes core strength and stability.

3. The Dead Bug Exercise: Despite its funny name, the dead bug exercise is an extremely effective method for strengthening the core and maintaining stability. While lying on their backs with their arms extended toward the ceiling and their legs up in a tabletop position,

persons alternately extend one arm overhead and the opposite leg towards the floor. This is done while keeping a stable pelvis and spine.

4. Bridge Stance: This yoga-inspired pose works the lower back, glutes, and hamstrings while also activating the core muscles for stability. It was inspired by yoga. Individuals elevate their hips toward the sky while lying on their backs with their knees bent and their feet hip-width apart. This creates a straight line from the shoulders to the knees through the entire body. A variety of variations, such as bridge with a stability ball or bridge with a single leg, provide a new dimension of difficulty and complexity to the workout.

5. One of the most well-known exercises in the Pilates repertoire, the Pilates Hundred is a combination of abdominal engagement and rhythmic arm motions that are designed to stress the core muscles and develop endurance. People perform this exercise while lying on their backs with their legs raised in a tabletop position. They pump their arms up and down while simultaneously working their abdominal muscles and keeping their spine in a neutral position.

By include these core strengthening techniques in their training routine, individuals have the opportunity to build the muscles that are necessary for maintaining stability, maintaining balance, and performing functional movements. It is possible for individuals to become better equipped to do daily activities with ease and confidence as their core muscles get stronger and more resilient. This, in turn, reduces the danger of falling and sustained injuries.

Cultivating Balance and Stability for Optimal Well-being

One of the most important aspects of physical fitness is the capacity to keep one's equilibrium and steadiness, which has an effect on every aspect of our individual lives. Through the incorporation of chair yoga poses, proprioception exercises, and core strengthening techniques into their daily routines, individuals have the opportunity to cultivate these key attributes. All things considered, this will lead to an improvement in their overall well-being as well as their quality of life. Through the cultivation of mindfulness, body awareness, and functional strength, individuals have the ability to empower themselves to navigate the challenges that life presents with grace, confidence, and vitality. As they embark on this journey of self-discovery and development, they begin to embrace equilibrium and steadiness as the foundations of their well-being. This allows them to go on a path that leads to optimal health and vitality as they make their way through this journey.

Chapter 6: Flexibility and Range of Motion

Flexibility and range of motion are essential components of overall health and well-being, and this is especially true for people who are in their senior years. As we get older, our muscles have a tendency to lose their flexibility, our joints become more rigid, and our range of motion may become more restricted. The flexibility and range of motion of senior citizens can be maintained and even improved through the use of joint mobilization techniques and stretching exercises on a regular basis. This will result in an improvement in the seniors' quality of life and a reduction in the likelihood of them suffering an injury. In addition, the incorporation of activities such as yoga can not only bring benefits to one's physical health but also contribute to one's mental and emotional well-being. Within the scope of this chapter, we will investigate moderate stretching exercises, joint mobilization techniques, and yoga postures that are specifically designed for older citizens in order to assist them in enhancing their flexibility and range of motion.

Gentle Stretching Exercises for Seniors:

1. Neck Stretch:

   - Take a tall stance or sit up straight with your shoulders relaxed.

   - In order to experience a slight stretch on the other side of your neck, slowly tilt your head to one side while bringing your ear closer to your shoulder. Continue this motion until you feel the stretch.

- After holding for fifteen to thirty seconds, switch sides.

- Do this two to three times on each side.

2. Shoulder Stretch:

- Stretch out one arm across your body until it is at shoulder level.

- You should feel a stretch in your shoulder and upper back as you bring the arm closer to your chest with the help of your other hand and gently press it there.

- After holding for fifteen to thirty seconds, switch sides.

- Do this two to three times on each side.

3. Chest Stretch:

- Your feet should be shoulder-width apart while you stand tall tall.

- Your arms should be straightened and your hands should be clasped behind your back.

- At the same time as you are lifting your hands slightly, squeeze your shoulder blades together.

- Focus on expanding up your chest and shoulders while you hold this position for fifteen to thirty seconds.

- Repeat 2-3 times.

4. Seated Forward Fold:

    - Sit on the edge of a chair with your feet flat on the floor.

    - Extend your arms overhead and lengthen your spine.

    - Slowly hinge forward at your hips, reaching your hands towards your feet or the floor.

    - Hold for 15-30 seconds, feeling a stretch along your spine and the back of your legs.

    - Repeat 2-3 times.

5. Quadriceps Stretch:

    - If you feel the need for support, stand close to a wall or a chair.

    - Bring your heel closer to your buttocks while bending one knee and grasping your ankle or foot with your hand. Now, bend the other knee.

    - Maintain a close knee-to-knee distance and an upright posture with your torso.

    - After holding for fifteen to thirty seconds, switch legs.

- Repeat 2-3 times on each side.

6. Hamstring Stretch:

    - Sit on the floor with one leg extended straight in front of you and the other bent with the sole of the foot against the inner thigh of the extended leg.

    - Reach forward towards your toes, keeping your back straight.

    - Hold for 15-30 seconds, feeling a stretch along the back of your thigh.

    - Switch legs and repeat.

    - Repeat 2-3 times on each side.

7. Calf Stretch:

    - Stand facing a wall with your hands resting on it for support.

    - Step one foot back and press the heel into the floor.

    - Keep the back leg straight and the front knee bent slightly.

    - Lean forward, feeling a stretch in the calf of the back leg.

    - Hold for 15-30 seconds, then switch legs.

    - Repeat 2-3 times on each side.

8. Ankle Circles:

    - Sit on a chair with your feet flat on the floor.

    - Lift one foot off the ground and rotate your ankle in a circular motion.

    - Perform 10 circles in one direction, then switch directions.

    - Repeat with the other foot.

    - Perform 2-3 sets on each side.

Joint Mobilization Techniques:

Through the use of gentle movements that take the joints through their range of motion, joint mobilization procedures are designed to increase the mobility of certain joints. The use of these strategies can assist in reducing stiffness, increasing flexibility, and providing relief from joint pain. For senior citizens, the following exercises are recommended for joint mobilization:

1. Shoulder Circles:

    - Stand tall with your arms relaxed at your sides.

    - Slowly roll your shoulders forward in a circular motion, making full rotations.

    - After 10 circles, reverse the direction and roll your shoulders backward.

    - Repeat for 2-3 sets.

2. Wrist Flexion and Extension:

- Sit or stand with your arms extended in front of you at shoulder height.

- Bend your wrists downward, pointing your fingers towards the floor, and hold for a few seconds.

- Then, bend your wrists upward, pointing your fingers towards the ceiling, and hold for a few seconds.

- Repeat for 10 repetitions.

3. Knee Extensions:

- Sit on a chair with your feet flat on the floor.

- Straighten one leg out in front of you, lifting your foot off the ground.

- Hold for a few seconds, then lower your foot back down.

- Repeat with the other leg.

- Perform 10 repetitions on each leg.

4. Ankle Alphabet:

- Sit on a chair with your feet hovering slightly above the ground.

- Pretend your big toe is a pen and write the alphabet in the air with your foot.

- Perform the entire alphabet with one foot, then switch to the other foot.

- Repeat for 2-3 sets on each foot.

5. Hip Circles:

- Stand with your feet hip-width apart and your hands on your hips.

- Slowly rotate your hips in a circular motion, making full rotations.

- After 10 circles in one direction, reverse the direction.

- Repeat for 2-3 sets.

Yoga Poses to Increase Flexibility:

Flexibility, strength, and relaxation are all benefits that can be gained from practicing yoga, which is a holistic practice that incorporates physical postures, breathwork, and meditation. As a result of their adaptability to the specific requirements and capabilities of each individual, several yoga poses are useful for senior citizens. For those looking to develop their flexibility, here are some gentle yoga poses:

1. Cat-Cow Stretch:

- To begin, assume a tabletop position on your hands and knees. Place your wrists so that they are aligned under your shoulders, and position your knees so that they are under your hips.

- By arching your back and drawing your chest and tailbone closer to the ceiling, you should take a deep breath (Cow Pose).

- You should exhale as you round your spine, bringing your belly button closer to your spine and tucking your chin into your chest (Cat Pose).

- For the next five to ten breaths, continue to flow between the Cat Pose and the Cow Pose, concentrating on syncing your movement with your breath.

2. Downward-Facing Dog:

   - Be in a tabletop position and begin by getting down on your hands and knees.

   - In order to create an inverted V shape, you need first tuck your toes under and then elevate your hips towards the ceiling. Your arms and legs should be straightened out.

   - Your hands should be firmly planted on the ground, your spine should be stretched out, and your heels should be drawn closer to the earth.

   - The spine should be lengthened and the backs of the legs should be opened while you hold this position for five to ten breaths.

3. Standing Forward Bend:

- Standing tall with your arms by your sides and your feet hip-width apart is the ideal position.

- Taking a deep breath, raise your arms above your head.

- Exhale as you tilt forward at the hips, bringing your hands towards the floor or resting them on your shins or thighs instead of bringing them to the floor.

- If necessary, bend your knees slightly in order to keep your spine in a straight position.

- For five to ten breaths, hold this position until you feel a stretch along the back of your legs and spine.

4. Seated Forward Bend

- Assume a seated position on the ground with your legs stretched out in front of you in a straight line and your feet bent.

- As you stretch your arms above your head and lengthen your spine, take a deep breath in.

- As you tilt forward at the hips and reach towards your feet or shins, exhale as you do so.

- It is important to avoid rounding your back and to maintain a straight spine.

- As you hold this position for five to ten breaths, you should feel a stretch running over the full length of your spine and the backs of your legs.

5. Warrior I:

    - Assume a standing position at the top of the mat with your feet equally spaced apart.

    - As you step your right foot back into a lunge position, maintain a 90-degree bend in your left knee during the entire movement.

    - At the same time that you are reaching your arms aloft with your palms facing each other, you should square your hips towards the front of the mat.

    - With a solid press through the outer border of your back foot, elevate your chest and press through your back foot.

    - When you feel a stretch in the hip flexors and chest, hold this position for five to ten breaths.

6. Warrior II:

    - To begin, open your hips toward the side of the mat and bring your back foot parallel to the back border of the mat. This is the first step in the Warrior I position.

- Make sure that your palms are facing down as you extend your arms out to the sides; they should be at shoulder height.

- In order to stack your front knee directly over your ankle, you should look over your front hand and bend your front knee.

- Maintain a comfortable posture with your shoulders and an open chest.

- Feel a stretch in the groin and side body as you hold this position for five to ten breaths.

7. Tree Pose:

- Standing tall with your arms by your sides and your feet hip-width apart is the ideal position.

- Your weight should be transferred to your left foot, and your right foot should be lifted off the ground.

- To avoid putting pressure on the knee joint, position the bottom of your right foot on the inside of your left thigh or calf at the same time.

- Bring both of your hands to the middle of your chest, or extend them above your head.

- Locate a focal point that will assist you in maintaining your balance and stability.

- Then, switch sides after holding for five to ten breaths.

8. Corpse Pose:

- Maintain a supine position with your legs stretched out in front of you and your arms by your sides, palms facing upward.

- Simply close your eyes and give your body the opportunity to thoroughly relax.

- Bring your attention to your breathing and allow it to become more calm and steady.

- As you hold this position for five to ten minutes, let go of any tension that you feel with each exhalation.

It is possible for seniors to greatly increase their flexibility and range of motion by including yoga postures, joint mobilization techniques, and mild stretching exercises into their daily routine. These practices not only contribute to the preservation of physical health, but they also encourage relaxation, the reduction of stress, and overall well-being throughout the body. In order to accommodate specific restrictions or injuries, it is vital to pay attention to your body and make adjustments to your workout routine as required. Senior citizens can reap the benefits of enhanced flexibility, increased mobility, and an overall improvement in their quality of life if they make a commitment to following a regular practice.

Chapter 7: Relaxation and Stress Reduction

Because of the fast-paced nature of the modern world, stress has become an unavoidable component of our lives. It is possible for stress to have a substantial influence on both our physical and emotional well-being, regardless of whether it is caused by strains at work, difficulties in personal relationships, worries about money, or health problems. The good news is that there are a variety of relaxation techniques that can assist us in efficiently managing stress and fostering a sense of calm and tranquility in our lives.

Within the scope of this chapter, we will investigate three effective methods of relaxation: guided relaxation, mindfulness meditation, and Yoga Nidra. It is possible to obtain profound relaxation and a reduction in stress by practicing any one of these techniques singly or in combination. Each of these techniques offers its own set of benefits.

Guided Relaxation Techniques

Through the process of following verbal instructions from a facilitator or listening to recorded audio, guided relaxation is a well-known technique that is used to induce a state of profound relaxation. Progressive muscle relaxation, breathing exercises, visualization, and other relaxation tactics are often included in this technique. The goal of this technique is to assist individuals in releasing tension and stress from their bodies and brains.

One of the most important advantages of guided relaxation is that it is easily accessible. It is possible to practice it nearly anywhere, which makes it perfect for people who have a lot going on in their lives or who might not have access to specific equipment or facilities. Participants are able to personalize their experience in order to achieve the highest possible level of relaxation and stress alleviation through the use of guided relaxation, which can be adapted to meet the preferences and requirements of each individual.

Finding a calm and comfortable place where you won't be interrupted is necessary in order to engage in the practice of guided relaxation. Put yourself in a relaxed position, either sitting or lying down, close your eyes, and concentrate on your breathing. The next step is to follow the instructions that are being guided, allowing yourself to completely submerge yourself in the experience and letting go of any tension or fears that you may have.

When you are working through the relaxation practice, it is important to pay attention to how your body and mind continue to react. Take note of any locations that are causing you discomfort or stress, and with each exhale, intentionally release those areas. Permit yourself to sink further into relaxation with each breath, and let go of any ideas or distractions that may come up during this process.

Individuals who battle with chronic stress, anxiety, or insomnia may find that guided relaxation is particularly beneficial to them. You may educate your body and mind to relax more deeply and readily by practicing relaxation techniques on a daily basis. This will result in greater sleep quality, decreased anxiety levels, and an overall improvement in your well-being.

Mindfulness Meditation

Mindfulness meditation is a practice that has been around for centuries and has its origins in Buddhist traditions. In recent years, it has gained widespread popularity due to the numerous health benefits it offers, including the reduction of stress, improvement of focus, and increased emotional resilience. Practitioners of mindfulness meditation are able to create a sense of clarity, acceptance, and inner calm by paying purposeful attention to the present moment without passing judgment on what they see or experience.

The awareness of one's breath is considered to be one of the most essential elements of mindfulness meditation. Make sure you are seated in a comfortable posture and close your eyes before beginning to practice this method. During the process of naturally inhaling and exhaling, bring your focus to your breath and pay attention to the feelings that the breath experiences as it enters and exits your body.

It is quite normal for your mind to wander while you continue to concentrate on your breath, and you may find that you become aware of this phenomenon. You should merely acknowledge your thoughts without passing judgment on them and then gently return your focus back to your breathing. This will prevent you from being frustrated or trying to repress your thoughts.

Not only is the practice of awareness of breath one of the many mindfulness meditation techniques that can assist promote relaxation and stress reduction, but there are also many other activities. Body scan meditations, loving-kindness meditations, and mindfulness meditations of thoughts or feelings are some examples of these types of meditations.

Meditations that incorporate body scans involve bringing awareness to various parts of the body in a methodical manner, observing any sensations or tension that may be there, and allowing them to soften and relax. Meditations designed to cultivate feelings of compassion and goodwill toward oneself and others are known as loving-kindness meditations. These meditations have the potential to assist in the reduction of unpleasant emotions such as stress, anger, or resentment.

Observing the contents of one's mind without becoming engrossed in them is an essential component in practicing mindfulness with regard to thought or emotion. This practise has the potential to assist individuals in developing better emotional awareness and resilience, which in turn enables them to respond more skillfully to tough situations and reduces their stress reactivity responses.

Practicing Yoga Nidra to Achieve Deep Calm

The powerful relaxation technique known as Yoga Nidra, which is also commonly referred to as yogic sleep, is a combination of components of meditation, guided imagery, and bodily awareness. Its purpose is to create a state of profound relaxation and regeneration throughout the practitioner. Since its inception in ancient yogic practices, Yoga Nidra has been increasingly popular in recent years due to its capacity to facilitate profound healing on all levels, including the physical, the mental, and the emotional.

Yoga Nidra is a form of meditation that, in contrast to traditional meditation methods, which include maintaining consciousness and focus, leads people into a state of profound relaxation that is dangerously close to sleep while still allowing them to stay consciously aware. Practitioners are able to access deeper areas of the subconscious mind, which is where great healing and transformation can take place, when they are in this state of conscious relaxation.

In order to practice Yoga Nidra, you will need to locate a place that is calm, comfortable, and that allows you to lie down without being disturbed. You should close your eyes and take a few moments to get into a peaceful position. This will help your body to relax and let go of any stress that may be associated with it. The next step is to participate in a guided Yoga Nidra meditation, which normally consists of a sequence of verbal instructions that are intended to guide you through various levels of relaxation and inner exploration.

During a normal session of Yoga Nidra, you may be directed to concentrate on sensations in the body, pay attention to the breath, picture images or symbols, or recite affirmations or sankalpas (positive intentions). The purpose of these instructions is to help you achieve a state of profound relaxation while simultaneously fostering self-awareness, helping you discover more about yourself, and facilitating inner healing.

The capacity of Yoga Nidra to induce significant transformation at the subconscious level is one of the distinctive features that distinguish it from other practices. Practitioners are able to identify and release deeply rooted patterns of stress, tension, and trauma by accessing the deepest layers of the mind. This results in increased emotional balance, mental clarity, and general well-being for the practitioner.

It has been demonstrated through research that regular practice of Yoga Nidra can have numerous positive effects on both physical and mental health. These benefits include a reduction in stress and anxiety, an improvement in the quality of sleep, an improvement in mood, and an increase in resilience to those who cause stress. In addition, Yoga Nidra has been utilized in therapeutic settings to assist participants in recovering from a variety of diseases, including addiction, chronic pain, and traumatic experiences.

It is possible to effectively manage stress, promote relaxation, and improve general well-being by employing relaxation techniques such as guided relaxation, mindfulness meditation, and Yoga Nidra. These approaches are known as potent tools. You can create more resilience, balance, and mental calm in the face of the obstacles that life presents to you by implementing these techniques into your daily routine. These methods, whether utilized singly or in conjunction with one another, have the ability to revolutionize your relationship with stress and assist you in leading a life that is more satisfying and enjoyable.

88

Chapter 8: Adapting Yoga for Special Conditions

Numerous medical disorders, such as osteoporosis, chronic pain, arthritis, and heart health problems, can be accommodated by yoga. People can benefit from increased physical comfort, mobility, and general well-being by tailoring yoga practices to address particular health issues and limits. Finding poses and methods that suit your body best is important, whether you're using chair yoga for arthritic relief, gentle yoga for osteoporosis, heart-healthy yoga for cardiovascular problems, or yoga for managing chronic pain. Yoga can be an effective technique for improving health and vitality at any age and stage of life if practiced with patience and attention.

Chair Yoga for Arthritis Relief

Inflammation and stiffness in the joints are characteristic symptoms of arthritis, which can greatly reduce mobility and quality of life. For those with arthritis, chair yoga provides a pleasant and convenient approach to reap the benefits of yoga with less strain on the joints.

Benefits of Chair Yoga for Arthritis Relief:

1. Gentle Movement: The emphasis of chair yoga is on stretches and mild motions that aid increase range of motion and joint flexibility without placing undue strain on the joints.

2. Improved Circulation: Practicing chair yoga can assist improve circulation, which helps reduce inflammation and facilitate healing in arthritic joints.

3. Pain management: By encouraging relaxation and releasing tension in the muscles surrounding the afflicted joints, specific yoga poses and breathing exercises can help reduce pain brought on by arthritis.

4. Enhanced Stability and Balance: Chair yoga incorporates stability and balance exercises that can help lower the chance of falls, which is a significant worry for people with arthritis.

5. Mind-Body Connection: Deep breathing exercises and meditation are examples of mindfulness techniques that are incorporated into chair yoga. These techniques can help people manage stress and feel better overall.

Adaptations for Chair Yoga:

- Seated Positions: You can modify a lot of the classic yoga poses to practice sitting down in a chair. For instance, you can perform sitting twists, forward folds, and mild stretches while seated.

- Use of Props: You can adjust poses and make them more accessible for people with restricted mobility or stiff joints by using props like blankets, harnesses, and blocks.

- Breathing Techniques: To induce relaxation and lower stress levels, sit in a chair and perform deep breathing techniques like diaphragmatic breathing and alternate nostril breathing.

- Mindfulness Techniques: People with arthritis can develop a better sense of awareness and acceptance of their bodies by incorporating mindfulness techniques like body scans and guided meditation.

Sample Chair Yoga Sequence for Arthritis Relief:

1. Seated Cat-Cow Stretch: Place your feet flat on the floor and sit tall on a chair. Breathe in, raise your chest, and arch your spine (Cow Pose). Breathe out, arch your back, and lower your chin to your chest (Cat Pose). Continue for a few breaths.

2. Forward-folded sitting position: Place your feet hip-width apart and lean toward the front of the chair. Exhale, bend forward from the hips, and reach for the floor or your feet. Inhale, lengthen your spine. Take a few deep breaths to hold, and then slowly raise yourself back up.

3. Sitting Spinal Twist: Place your feet flat on the ground and sit tall on the chair. Breathe in, lengthening your spine; then, exhale and twist to the right, resting your right hand on the chair's back and your left hand on your right knee. After holding for a few breaths, switch to the other side and repeat.

4. Chair Pigeon Pose: With your feet flat on the ground, sit tall in the chair. Flex the right foot by crossing the right ankle over the left knee. Feel the stretch in your right hip and glute as you slowly bend forward while maintaining a long spine. After holding for a few breaths, switch to the other side and repeat.

5. For seated meditation, place your feet flat on the ground and find a comfortable seat. Shut your eyes and focus on your breathing, taking slow, deep breaths in and out. Take a few minutes to practice quiet meditation, paying attention to your body's sensations and letting your ideas come and go without judgment.

Yoga for Osteoporosis

Osteoporosis is a condition characterized by weakened bones, making them more susceptible to fractures and breaks. Yoga can be a beneficial practice for individuals with osteoporosis, as it can help improve bone density, balance, and flexibility while reducing the risk of falls and fractures.

Benefits of Yoga for Osteoporosis:

1. **Bone Health: In order to maintain strong and healthy bones, weight-bearing yoga poses help promote bone growth and density.**

2. **Strengthening your muscles is essential for maintaining bone health and lowering your chance of falling. Yoga poses that work on your legs, hips, spine, and core can help you do this.**

3. **Balance and Coordination:** Yoga poses that emphasize balance and coordination can help increase stability and lower the chance of falls. This is especially beneficial for people who have osteoporosis, as they may be more susceptible to fractures.

4. **Posture Alignment:** By enhancing spinal health and posture alignment, yoga can lower the incidence of compression fractures and other osteoporosis-related spine problems.

5. **Stress Reduction:** People with osteoporosis can manage stress and feel better overall by including mindfulness techniques like meditation and deep breathing into their yoga practice.

Adaptations for Yoga for Osteoporosis:

- **Steer Clear of Forward Bends:** People who have osteoporosis should steer clear of forward bends that require flexing their spines because they raise the risk of compression fractures. Rather, concentrate on lateral stretches and mild backbends that enhance spinal health and posture.

- **Employ Props for Support:** Yoga poses can be made more accessible for people with osteoporosis by using props like blankets, straps, and blocks to offer stability and support.

- **Concentrate on Poses That Build Strength:** Exercises that concentrate on the muscles of the hips, back, legs, and core can enhance general muscle stability and strength, which is beneficial for maintaining bone health and lowering the risk of fractures.

- **Exercises for Balance Practice:** Include balancing exercises to increase stability and lower the chance of falling, such as warrior III, tree pose, and standing leg lifts.

Sample Yoga Sequence for Osteoporosis:

1. **Mountain Pose (Tadasana):** Stand tall with feet hip-width apart, arms by your sides. Engage the muscles of the legs and core, and lengthen through the spine. Hold for several breaths, focusing on grounding through the feet and lifting through the crown of the head.

2. **Warrior II (Virabhadrasana II):** From Mountain Pose, step the feet wide apart. Turn the right foot out 90 degrees and the left foot in slightly. Bend the right knee, stacking it directly over the right ankle. Extend the arms out parallel to the floor, gaze over the right fingertips. Hold for several breaths, then switch sides.

3. **Tree Pose (Vrksasana):** Stand tall with feet hip-width apart. Shift weight onto the left foot and lift the right foot, placing the sole against the inner left thigh or calf. Press the foot into the thigh or calf and engage the muscles of the standing leg. Bring hands to prayer

position at the heart or extend arms overhead. Hold for several breaths, then switch sides.

4. **Bridge Pose (Setu Bandhasana)**: Lie on your back with knees bent and feet hip-width apart. Press into the feet and lift the hips towards the ceiling, engaging the glutes and thighs. Interlace the fingers beneath the body and roll the shoulders underneath. Hold for several breaths, then release slowly back to the floor.

5. **Seated Forward Fold**: Sit on the floor with legs extended in front of you. Inhale, lengthen the spine, and exhale, hinge forward from the hips, reaching towards the feet or the floor. Hold for several breaths, then slowly return to an upright position.

Yoga for Heart Health

Although heart disease is one of the major causes of mortality worldwide, practicing yoga can help to maintain heart health and lower the risk of cardiovascular problems. Practices of yoga that emphasize mindfulness, gentle movement, and stress reduction can help people manage risk factors like high blood pressure, high cholesterol, and stress.

Benefits of Yoga for Heart Health:

1. **Stress Reduction: People can manage their stress and lower their chance of heart disease by including**

mindfulness techniques like deep breathing and meditation into their yoga practice.

2. **Enhanced Circulation:** Breathing exercises and some yoga poses can assist enhance circulation, which is important for heart health and lowering the risk of cardiovascular problems.

3. **Reduce Blood Pressure:** Research has indicated that regular yoga practice can help reduce blood pressure, a major risk factor for heart disease.

4. **Improved Flexibility and Range of Motion:** By encouraging improved circulation and cardiovascular function, gentle yoga poses can assist increase the flexibility and range of motion in the muscles and joints, which can benefit general heart health.

5. **Weight Management:** Controlling weight is another crucial component in avoiding heart disease and preserving general health. Yoga can be a useful technique in this regard.

Adaptations for Yoga for Heart Health:

- **Emphasis on Gentle Movement:** For people who are concerned about their heart health, gentle yoga practices that emphasize slow, controlled motions are perfect. Steer clear of demanding or stressful activities that could raise your blood pressure or heart rate.

- **Include Breathing Exercises:** Deep breathing techniques that lower blood pressure, increase relaxation, and reduce stress include diaphragmatic and alternate nostril breathing.

- **Practice Mindfulness Meditation:** To assist lower stress, enhance emotional well-being, and support heart health, incorporate mindfulness meditation into your yoga practice.

- **Pay Attention to Your Body:** During your yoga practice, pay attention to how your body feels and refrain from pushing yourself over your comfort zone. Stop and relax if you feel any pain or lightheadedness.

Sample Yoga Sequence for Heart Health:

1. **Easy Seated Pose (Sukhasana):** Sit comfortably on the floor or in a chair with legs crossed and hands resting on the knees. Close the eyes and bring attention to the breath, inhaling and exhaling slowly and deeply. Hold for several breaths, focusing on relaxation and stress reduction.

2. **Cat-Cow Stretch:** Come to a tabletop position on hands and knees. Inhale, arch the back, and lift the chest (Cow Pose). Exhale, round the spine, and tuck the chin towards the chest (Cat Pose). Repeat for several breaths, moving with the rhythm of the breath.

3. **Child's Pose (Balasana):** From tabletop position, sit back on the heels and lower the forehead to the mat, extending the arms forward or resting them by the

sides. Relax into the pose, breathing deeply into the back body. Hold for several breaths, allowing the body to soften and release tension.

4. **Seated Forward Fold**: Sit on the floor with legs extended in front of you. Inhale, lengthen the spine, and exhale, hinge forward from the hips, reaching towards the feet or the floor. Hold for several breaths, focusing on lengthening the spine and releasing tension in the hamstrings and lower back.

5. **Corpse Pose (Savasana)**: Lie on your back with legs extended and arms by your sides, palms facing up. Close the eyes and allow the body to relax completely, releasing tension in the muscles and letting go of any stress or worries. Remain in Savasana for several minutes, focusing on deep relaxation and rejuvenation.

Yoga for Chronic Pain Management

Chronic pain is a complex condition that can have a significant impact on physical and emotional well-being. While yoga may not offer a cure for chronic pain, it can be a valuable tool for managing symptoms and improving quality of life by promoting relaxation, reducing stress, and increasing body awareness.

Benefits of Yoga for Chronic Pain Management:

1. Pain Relief: By reducing muscle tension, enhancing circulation, and encouraging relaxation, specific yoga

positions and breathing exercises can help reduce chronic pain.

2. Increased Flexibility: Moderate yoga poses can assist increase range of motion and flexibility in the muscles and joints, which can help lessen stiffness and pain related to long-term pain issues.

3. Stress Reduction: People can manage stress and lessen their perception of pain by including mindfulness techniques like deep breathing and meditation into their yoga practice.

4. Enhanced Body Awareness: Yoga teaches practitioners to tune into their bodies and become more conscious of their sensations, which can improve their comprehension and management of pain.

5. Enhanced Emotional Well-Being: By encouraging relaxation, lowering anxiety and sadness, and elevating emotions of serenity and contentment, yoga can help enhance emotional well-being.

Adaptations for Yoga for Chronic Pain Management:

- Listen to Your Body: During your yoga practice, be aware of how your body is feeling. Adjust the poses accordingly to prevent aggravating any pain or discomfort.

- Emphasis on Gentle Movement: People with chronic pain disorders benefit greatly from gentle yoga practices that emphasize calm, controlled movements. Steer clear of demanding or taxing activities that could make pain worse.

- Employ Props for Support: Yoga poses can be made more accessible and comfortable for people with chronic pain by using props like blankets, straps, and blocks to offer stability and support.

- Incorporate Methods of Relaxation: To assist lower tension, encourage relaxation, and ease discomfort, incorporate relaxation techniques including progressive muscle relaxation, deep breathing, and guided imagery.

Sample Yoga Sequence for Chronic Pain Management:

1. **Seated Neck Stretch**: Sit tall in a chair with feet flat on the floor. Inhale, lengthen the spine, and exhale, drop the right ear towards the right shoulder, feeling a stretch in the left side of the neck. Hold for several breaths, then switch sides.

2. **Cat-Cow Stretch**: Come to a tabletop position on hands and knees. Inhale, arch the back, and lift the chest (Cow Pose). Exhale, round the spine, and tuck the chin towards the chest (Cat Pose). Repeat for several breaths, moving with the rhythm of the breath.

3. **Supported Child's Pose**: Place a bolster or stack of blankets on the mat. Kneel on the floor and place the bolster or blankets between the thighs. Sit back on the heels and lower the forehead to the support, extending the arms forward or resting them by the sides. Relax

into the pose, breathing deeply into the back body. Hold for several breaths, allowing the body to soften and release tension.

4. **Supported Bridge Pose**: Lie on your back with knees bent and feet hip-width apart. Place a block or bolster beneath the sacrum and lower back. Press into the feet and lift the hips towards the ceiling, engaging the glutes and thighs. Allow the body to relax into the support. Hold for several breaths, then release slowly back to the floor.

5. **Corpse Pose (Savasana)**: Lie on your back with legs extended and arms by your sides, palms facing up. Close the eyes and allow the body to relax completely, releasing tension in the muscles and letting go of any stress or worries. Remain in Savasana for several minutes, focusing on deep relaxation and rejuvenation.

Yoga can be modified to accommodate a wide range of particular diseases, such as osteoporosis, arthritis, heart health difficulties, and chronic pain, among others. It is possible for individuals to enjoy greater physical comfort, mobility, and overall well-being by adapting yoga practices in order to meet specific health challenges and limits. No matter if you are practicing chair yoga for the relief of arthritis, gentle yoga for osteoporosis, heart-healthy yoga for cardiovascular issues, or yoga for the management of chronic pain, the most important thing is to pay attention to your body, incorporate mindfulness into your practice, and find the movements and techniques that are most effective for you. Yoga has the potential to be an effective method for boosting health and vitality at any age and stage of life, provided that it is practiced with dedication and patience.

Chapter 9: Yoga Philosophy and Lifestyle

Yoga, which has its roots in ancient India, is not only a physical practice; rather, it is an all-encompassing philosophy for holistic well-being that encompasses the body, the mind, and the soul. The Eight Limbs, which are described in Patanjali's Yoga Sutras, are considered to be the most important aspect of the yoga philosophy. In addition to fostering self-awareness, self-discipline, and spiritual development, these limbs serve as guides for living a life that is personally meaningful and rewarding. Throughout this chapter, we will investigate the Eight Limbs of Yoga, look into the various ways in which yogic concepts can be incorporated into daily life, and talk about the significance of cultivating appreciation and mindfulness.

Understanding the Eight Limbs of Yoga

1. **Yamas (Restraints)**: The Yamas are ethical principles guiding our interactions with the world around us. They consist of:

   - **Ahimsa (Non-violence)**: Practicing kindness and compassion towards oneself and others.

   - **Satya (Truthfulness)**: Being honest in thoughts, speech, and actions.

   - **Asteya (Non-stealing)**: Respecting the possessions and boundaries of others.

   - **Brahmacharya (Moderation)**: Exercising control over our senses and desires.

- **Aparigraha (Non-possessiveness)**: Letting go of greed and attachment to material possessions.

2. **Niyamas (Observances)**: The Niyamas are personal observances focused on self-discipline and inner growth. They include:

   - **Saucha (Cleanliness)**: Maintaining cleanliness of body, mind, and environment.

   - **Santosha (Contentment)**: Cultivating gratitude for what we have and finding peace within.

   - **Tapas (Discipline)**: Practicing self-discipline and perseverance to achieve goals.

   - **Svadhyaya (Self-study)**: Engaging in self-reflection, study, and introspection.

   - **Ishvara Pranidhana (Surrender to a higher power)**: Letting go of ego and surrendering to the divine.

3. **Asanas (Postures)**: Asanas are physical postures practiced in yoga to promote strength, flexibility, and balance. They prepare the body for meditation and cultivate mindfulness.

4. **Pranayama (Breath Control)**: Pranayama involves breath control techniques aimed at regulating the breath, calming the mind, and increasing prana (life force energy) within the body.

5. **Pratyahara (Withdrawal of the Senses)**: Pratyahara is the practice of withdrawing the senses from external stimuli and turning the focus inward, facilitating meditation and self-awareness.

6. **Dharana (Concentration)**: Dharana is the practice of single-pointed concentration, focusing the mind on a particular object, mantra, or breath to cultivate mental clarity and stability.

7. **Dhyana (Meditation)**: Dhyana is the state of sustained focus and awareness, leading to a deep sense of inner peace, clarity, and transcendence of the self.

8. **Samadhi (Union with the Divine)**: Samadhi is the ultimate goal of yoga, a state of complete absorption where the practitioner experiences union with the divine and transcends the limitations of the ego.

Incorporating Yogic Principles into Daily Life

On the mat is where most people begin their yoga practice; nevertheless, the actual core of yoga rests in its application in our everyday life, which takes place away from the mat. The following are some examples of how yogic ideas can be incorporated into everyday life:

1. Cultivate mindfulness by being fully present in each moment, whether you are eating, walking, or having a conversation. This will help you cultivate mindfulness. Without passing judgment on your ideas, feelings, and sensations, pay attention to their presence.

2. Putting Ahimsa into practice is making a conscious decision to treat other people with compassion and kindness. Be conscious of the effect that your words and actions have on the people around you, and make it your goal to avoid causing any harm.

3. Truly live your life by adhering to the principles of honesty and integrity in every facet of your existence. In order to connect your activities with your values and beliefs, you should be truthful to both yourself and to other people.

4. Embrace the idea of Aparigraha by letting go of attachments to material possessions and outcomes. Simplify and let go of attachments. Reduce the amount of clutter in your environment and give priority to the things that are actually important to you.

5. Encourage Thankfulness: One way to put Santosha into practice is to encourage gratitude for all of the benefits in your life, no matter how great or how tiny. You can either keep a thankfulness book or simply take a moment every day to think about the things for which you are grateful.

6. Fostering Self-Reflection: Make time in your schedule for self-reflection and introspection, whether you do so through contemplative practices such as journaling, meditation, or other similar activities. Take use of this time to gain a deeper understanding of yourself and the world that is within you.

7. Serving Others: Seva, also known as selfless service, is a form of service that involves offering your time, skills, or resources to assist those who are in need. Being of service to other people not only benefits them, but it also provides them a sense of fulfillment and a connection to others.

8. Cultivate Balance: Strive to achieve a state of equilibrium in all aspects of your life, including but not limited to work and rest, activity and stillness, and socializing and seclusion. As much as you should respect your body's desire for movement and activity, you should also respect its need for rest and rejuvenation.

9. Spend time outside and establish a connection with the natural world by spending time in their company. Being in nature, whether it be through activities such as gardening, going for a stroll in the park, or simply sitting beneath a tree, can assist you in becoming more grounded and cultivating a sense of serenity and harmony.

10. Take Care of Yourself: Make it a priority to engage in self-care activities that provide nourishment to your body, mind, and spirit. This may include engaging in things that bring you joy and relaxation, as well as eating healthily, exercise on a regular basis, and getting enough rest.

11. Develop the ability to forgive: Exercise forgiveness, not only toward oneself but also toward other people. In order to liberate yourself from the burden of previous injuries and make room for healing and progress, it is important to let go of resentment, grudges, and bad emotions.

12. Live your life with purpose: You should live your life with purpose and intentionality, making sure that your actions are in line with your goals and ideals. Establish goals that are significant to you, and then work with determination and focus to move forward in the direction of achieving those goals.

Cultivating Gratitude and Mindfulness

There are two important disciplines that have the potential to radically improve our lives and our perspectives: gratitude and mindfulness. The practice of cultivating gratitude comprises acknowledging and appreciating the wealth that it brings into our lives, whereas the practice of mindfulness involves being completely present and aware in each moment. In your day-to-day existence, you can build thankfulness and mindfulness by applying the following strategies:

1. **Gratitude Practices**:

   - Maintaining a thankfulness diary involves devoting a few minutes of your time each day to writing down three things for which you are thankful. This easy technique has the potential to change your emphasis from what is missing in your life to what is abundant in your life.

- Verbalize your thanks: Make it a point to convey your gratitude to the people in your immediate environment, including friends, family, coworkers, and even complete strangers. One's day can be made better and connections can be strengthened with a simple expression of gratitude.

- A meditation practice based on gratitude: Set aside a few minutes of your time every day to engage in a practice of thankfulness meditation. Relax in a quiet place, bring your attention to your breathing, and think on the things for which you are thankful. Savor the sensations of gratitude and abundance that you experience.

2. **Mindfulness Practices**:

- In order to practice mindful breathing, you should pause for a few seconds during the day and concentrate on your breathing. While you are allowing yourself to come into the present now, pay attention to the sensations that accompany each inhale and exhale.

- In order to increase awareness of physical sensations and to induce relaxation, it is beneficial to practice a meditation technique known as body scan meditation. You should begin by focusing your attention on your toes and gradually move it up through your body, paying attention to any areas of tension or discomfort with an attitude of appreciation and curiosity.

- Take your time and relish each mouthful of your meals while practicing mindful eating. Pay attention to the flavors, textures, and sensations that you experience while you are eating. Enjoying food more and developing healthy eating habits are two benefits that might result from practicing mindful eating.

- Mindfully engaging in daily activities: To include mindfulness into your daily routine, whether you are walking, brushing your teeth, or doing the dishes, try adopting a thoughtful attitude. It is possible to bring mindfulness to even the most monotonous chores by approaching each task with complete concentration and awareness.

You can build a better sense of serenity, fulfillment, and connection with yourself and the world around you by adopting these practices into your everyday life and making them a part of your routine. For those who are interested in living a life that is purposeful, honest, and in accordance with themselves, yoga philosophy provides both timeless wisdom and practical assistance.

We are led on a path of self-discovery, self-awareness, and spiritual development by the Eight Limbs of Yoga, which provide a comprehensive framework for living a life that is meaningful and rewarding. Through the practice of cultivating gratitude and mindfulness, as well as implementing yogic principles into our daily lives, we are able to tap into the transformational potential of yoga and generate more harmony, balance, and well-being not just within ourselves but also within the world. When we embrace these practices with an open mind and a strong commitment, we bring a more profound connection, joy, and fulfillment into our life, and in the end, we come to realize the true essence of yoga both on and off the mat.

Chapter 10: Nutrition and Wellness Tips

In this chapter, we will delve into essential aspects of nutrition and wellness, particularly tailored for seniors. As we age, our bodies undergo various changes, making it crucial to adopt healthy eating habits, prioritize hydration, and cultivate positive lifestyle habits to maintain overall well-being.

Healthy Eating for Seniors

As we age, our nutritional needs evolve, necessitating adjustments to our dietary habits. Healthy eating for seniors entails a balanced diet rich in essential nutrients while being mindful of calorie intake to maintain a healthy weight. Here are some key considerations:

1. The consumption of nutrient-dense meals should be a top priority for senior citizens in order to fulfill their dietary requirements without consuming an excessive amount of calories. A sufficient amount of fruits, vegetables, whole grains, lean meats, and healthy fats are included in this consumption. In order to maintain maximum health, it is crucial to consume meals that include critical vitamins, minerals, and antioxidants.

2. Calcium and vitamin D: The risk of bone-related disorders such as osteoporosis grows with age. One of these diseases is osteoporosis. In order to maintain healthy bones, senior citizens should make sure they consume a proper amount of calcium and vitamin D. There are several excellent sources of these nutrients,

including dairy products, foods that have been fortified, leafy greens, and fatty fish.

3. It is essential to consume protein in order to preserve muscular mass and strength, both of which tend to decrease with decreasing age. It is recommended that senior citizens incorporate foods that are high in protein into their diet. These foods include lean meats, poultry, fish, eggs, beans, lentils, and dairy products.

4. Dietary fiber is beneficial for digestion, aids in the prevention of constipation, and contributes to the maintenance of good cholesterol levels. Whole grains, fruits, vegetables, nuts, and seeds are all examples of foods that are high in fiber and should be consumed by senior citizens in order to maintain digestive health.

5. Hydration: senior citizens are more likely to suffer from dehydration, which can result in a variety of health concerns. Drinking a proper amount of water throughout the day and consuming foods that are high in water content, such as fruits, vegetables, soups, and herbal teas, are both crucial parts of a healthy lifestyle.

6. Reduce Your Intake of Salt and Sugar: Consuming an excessive amount of sodium and sugar can contribute to several health problems, including high blood pressure, heart disease, and other conditions. The use of processed foods, canned soups, salty snacks, sugary drinks, and sweets needs to be reduced as much as possible for senior citizens.

7. Meals That Are Smaller and More Frequent: It may be good for senior citizens to consume meals that are smaller and more frequent rather than huge meals in order to facilitate digestion and sustain energy levels throughout the day.

8. By paying attention to indicators that indicate when you are hungry and when you are full, mindful eating can help prevent overeating and promote healthier eating habits. Seniors should make it a priority to enjoy their meals without interruptions and to take the time to appreciate the various flavors and textures of the food they eat.

9. Dietary supplements: In certain circumstances, elderly people may be required to take dietary supplements in order to treat particular nutritional deficits. Nevertheless, prior to beginning any supplementation regimen, it is absolutely necessary to discuss the matter with a qualified medical practitioner.

10. Having fun and interacting with others: The eating experience of older citizens can be improved by increasing the amount of social contact and emotional well-being that occurs when they have meals with their family and friends. Additionally, if they are interested in adding excitement and variety to their diet, they could try out different recipes and cuisines.

By incorporating these principles into their daily routine, seniors can maintain optimal nutrition and support overall health and well-being as they age.

Hydration Importance

Proper hydration is vital for everyone, but it holds particular significance for seniors due to age-related changes in the body's water balance and thirst perception. Here's why hydration is essential for seniors:

1. Temperature Regulation: Adequate hydration helps regulate body temperature, which helps prevent overheating or illnesses associated to heat, particularly when the weather is hot or when one is engaging in physical activity.

2. Lubrication of the Joints: Hydration has a role in maintaining joint health by ensuring appropriate lubrication, which helps decrease stiffness and discomfort, particularly in persons who suffer from arthritis or other joint issues.

3. Water is necessary for effective digestion and the absorption of nutrients, which is crucial for digestive health. When it comes to constipation and digestive disorders, senior citizens who drink plenty of water are less prone to have them.

4. Cognitive Function Dehydration can have a negative impact on cognitive function, which can result in issues such as confusion, inadequate focus, and memory problems. In order to preserve mental clarity and

cognitive health, it is essential to drink plenty of water, particularly for people who are getting older.

5. Intake of an adequate amount of fluids is beneficial to kidney function because it makes it easier for the kidneys to eliminate waste products and toxins from the body. When it comes to their hydration levels, senior citizens who have kidney function that is affected should pay additional care.

6. Heart Health: Adequate hydration helps to maintain blood volume and improves cardiovascular function, which in turn reduces the risk of issues associated to the heart, such as high blood pressure and heart disease.

7. When it comes to maintaining the skin's suppleness, elasticity, and hydration, proper hydration is absolutely necessary. When skin is dehydrated, it is more likely to experience dryness, flakiness, and wrinkles, all of which can make age-related skin problems even worse.

8. Dehydration can cause feelings of exhaustion, irritation, and poor energy levels, even in mild cases. This can have an effect on mood as well as energy levels. It is more likely that senior citizens who are well hydrated will have feelings of alertness, vigor, and be in a happy attitude.

To ensure proper hydration, seniors should aim to drink an adequate amount of fluids throughout the day, even if they don't feel thirsty. Water is the best choice, but other hydrating options include herbal teas, broth-based soups, fruits, and vegetables with high water content. It's essential to monitor urine color, as pale yellow urine indicates proper hydration, while dark urine may signal dehydration.

Lifestyle Habits for Overall Well-being

In addition to nutrition and hydration, adopting positive lifestyle habits is essential for promoting overall well-being in seniors. Here are some lifestyle tips:

1. Participating in regular physical activity is essential for preserving our mobility, strength, and flexibility as we get older. A wide range of activities, including walking, swimming, yoga, tai chi, and strength training exercises, should be participated in by senior citizens in order to preserve their physical health and maintain their independence.

2. When it comes to both physical and mental health, getting enough quality sleep is absolutely necessary. Seniors should strive to get between seven and nine hours of quality sleep every night. They should also practice good sleep hygiene habits, such as keeping a regular sleep schedule, developing a relaxing bedtime routine, and making sure that their sleeping environment is comfortable while they are sleeping.

3. Management of Stress: Prolonged exposure to stress can have negative consequences for one's health, including the exacerbation of a number of age-related illnesses. Research suggests that senior citizens should

investigate methods of stress reduction, such as practicing mindfulness meditation, deep breathing exercises, progressive muscle relaxation, or participating in activities and hobbies that they like.

4. Social Connection: It is essential for both emotional well-being and cognitive health to maintain social connections and to participate in activities that are relevant to relationships with other people. It is important for senior citizens to look for opportunities to connect with friends, family members, and community groups. These connections can be made through in-person get-togethers, phone calls, or internet interactions.

5. It is vital for cognitive function and mental clarity to maintain a state of brain stimulation, which involves keeping the brain active and stimulated. Seniors have the opportunity to participate in a variety of activities, including reading, puzzles, crossword puzzles, learning new skills or languages, playing musical instruments, and taking part in educational classes or workshops.

6. Regular Health Checkups: Seniors should make it a priority to get routine health screenings and checkups in order to maintain their overall health status and identify any potential problems at an earlier stage. Visits to medical specialists on a regular basis for the purpose of obtaining physical examinations, monitoring of blood pressure, blood tests, eye examinations, dental

checkups, and immunizations are included in this routine.

7. Healthy Relationships: Developing healthy relationships with members of one's family, friends, and caretakers not only provides emotional support but also improves one's general well-being. Open communication, the expression of wants and sentiments, and the seeking of support when it is required are all important for senior citizens.

8. Having a feeling of purpose and meaning in one's life is critical to one's mental and emotional health, and it is crucial to maintain this sense throughout one's life. There are a variety of activities, hobbies, volunteer opportunities, and personal goals that senior citizens should identify in order to achieve a sense of contentment and success.

At the same time that they are navigating the process of aging, older citizens can improve their physical health, emotional well-being, and general quality of life by implementing these lifestyle practices into their daily routine.

For the purpose of improving health and wellness in older citizens, it is essential to place diet, hydration, and beneficial lifestyle habits at the forefront of one's priorities. The adoption of a well-balanced diet that is abundant in essential nutrients, the maintenance of a healthy level of hydration, and the cultivation of habits that support physical, mental, and emotional well-being are all ways in which senior citizens can enjoy a life that is both fulfilling and vibrant as they age gently.

Chapter 11: Progress Tracking and Journaling

When it comes to the journey of practicing chair yoga, keeping a notebook and measuring your progress are two tools that are quite helpful. Not only do they assist in the process of goal-setting and goal-attainment, but they also offer insights into the physical and mental well-being of an individual. The importance of developing goals for chair yoga practice, keeping a daily notebook for reflection and growth, and keeping track of improvements in both physical and mental well-being is discussed in depth in this chapter.

Setting Goals for Chair Yoga Practice

The practice of chair yoga is no exception to the rule that setting goals is essential to any activity. A sense of success, as well as direction and inspiration, can be gained from setting goals. In the process of establishing objectives for chair yoga practice, it is vital to take into consideration both short-term and long-term goals.

Short-term Goals:

1. Your goal should be to practice chair yoga on a consistent basis, preferably on a daily basis or multiple times per week. Maintaining a consistent yoga practice helps to create momentum and brings about additional advantages.

2. In order to enhance your flexibility, you should establish goals to improve your flexibility in particular parts of your body, such as your spine, shoulders, and hips. As you engage in consistent practice, you will gradually observe gains in your range of motion and general mobility.

3. The relaxing effects that chair yoga has on the mind are well-known for their ability to reduce stress. By engaging in consistent practice, you can establish objectives to lower your levels of stress and build a sense of serenity and relaxation.

4. Enhancing Posture: A significant number of chair yoga postures are centered on enhancing body alignment and posture. In order to alleviate any discomfort or pain that may be related with bad posture, you should establish goals to improve your posture.

5. Even though chair yoga is a light kind of exercise, it can nevertheless be beneficial for growing strength, particularly in the abdominal region, the legs, and the uppermost part of the body. With the help of specific workouts, you should establish objectives to progressively improve your strength and stability.

Long-term Goals:

1. Learning More Advanced Pose Sequences and Pose Sequences As you become more proficient in your chair yoga practice, you may have the desire to learn more advanced poses and sequences. You should challenge

yourself and investigate new opportunities by setting long-term goals for yourself.

2. Improvements in Physical Fitness, Mental Clarity, and Emotional Balance Chair yoga helps to maintain total health by enhancing physical fitness, mental clarity, and emotional equilibrium. If you want to continue your profession while maintaining your ideal health and vigor, you need set goals.

3. In the event that you have a strong interest in chair yoga, you might want to think about establishing objectives to either become a certified instructor or to share your skills with other people. Through teaching, you can strengthen your practice while also having a beneficial impact on the lives of others, which can be a very satisfying experience.

When setting goals, it's crucial to make them specific, measurable, achievable, relevant, and time-bound (SMART). Write down your goals and revisit them regularly to track your progress and make any necessary adjustments.

Daily Reflection and Progress Journal

A daily reflection and progress journal is a powerful tool for self-awareness and personal growth. It provides a space for introspection, gratitude, and tracking your journey with chair yoga. Here's how to create and maintain a daily journal:

Determine the Format: Determine if you would like to keep a digital diary, a notepad, or an app that is specifically designed for journaling. It is important to select a format that is both comfortable and convenient for you.

Dedicate a Specific Time: Each day, pick a specific time to write in your diary, such as first thing in the morning or right before you go to bed. The key to successfully creating a habit is consistency.

Reflect on Your Practice: At the beginning of each writing in your journal, you should offer some thoughts about your chair yoga practice for the day. You should make a note of any realizations, difficulties, or breakthroughs that you had during your practice session.

Express Thanks: Take a moment to express gratitude for the chance to practice chair yoga as well as for any wonderful experiences or blessings that have occurred in your life.

The fifth step is to establish your intentions or affirmations for the day that lies ahead. During your practice and throughout your life, what are some qualities that you would like to cultivate?

Record any changes or improvements you've observed in your flexibility, strength, posture, or overall well-being. This is our sixth and last step in tracking your progress. Honor your accomplishments, no matter how insignificant they may seem.

Monitor Challenges: During your practice, you should acknowledge any difficulties or roadblocks that presented themselves to you. Think about the ways in which you can triumph over them and become more powerful as a result.

Encourage the cultivation of self-compassion by treating yourself with kindness, particularly on days when your practice appears to be difficult or does not meet your expectations. Develop a compassionate attitude toward oneself and keep in mind that making development takes time.

Reassess and Modify Your Goals It is important to regularly reassess your goals and evaluate how far you have come in the direction of accomplishing them. Do you need to make any adjustments or revisions in order to continue on the path that you have chosen?

Remain Consistent: Include journaling as a regular component of your chair yoga practice whenever possible. With the passage of time, you will accumulate a priceless record of your journey and acquire a more profound understanding of who you are.

Monitoring Changes in Physical and Mental Well-being
Chair yoga practice has numerous benefits for both physical and mental well-being. By monitoring changes in these areas, you can gain valuable insights into the effectiveness of your practice and make any necessary adjustments. Here are some key aspects to monitor:

Physical Well-being:

1. Flexibility: Take note of any potential enhancements in your range of motion and flexibility, particularly in areas such as the spine, shoulders, and hips. Is it

possible for you to move more easily and with less resistance?

2. Strength: Pay note to any increases in strength, especially in the abdominal region, the legs, and the upper body. In your chair yoga positions, do you experience a greater sense of stability and grounding?

3. Be aware of any shifts in your posture and alignment, and pay attention to them. You appear to be sitting more upright and with greater ease. Have you noticed a reduction in the amount of tension or soreness in your back, collarbone, or shoulders?

4. Track your progress in terms of your general mobility and your capacity to carry out activities of daily living with a greater degree of ease and grace. Are your movements becoming more fluid and requiring less effort?

Mental Well-being:

1. Stress Levels: Take note of any decreases in your stress levels as well as an increase in your sense of peace and relaxation. Are you experiencing a greater sense of focus and equilibrium in your day-to-day life?

2. Mental Clarity: Pay note to any increases in your mental clarity, focus, and concentration that you may experience. Are you able to gain a clearer understanding of the situation and make judgments with greater ease?

3. Observe any improvements in your emotional well-being, such as an increased sense of inner calm, joy, or resilience in the face of adversities. This is an important aspect of emotional balance. Are you experiencing a greater sense of emotional equilibrium and well-being?

If you routinely evaluate changes in your physical and emotional well-being, you will be able to obtain useful insights into the impact that your chair yoga practice has on your overall health and happiness. Keep in mind that change may occur gradually and in increments; therefore, it is important to be patient with yourself and have faith in the process.

In conclusion, there are two important components that are necessary for a good chair yoga practice: measuring progress and keeping a notebook. You may develop your practice, grow self-awareness, and experience improved health and vitality by setting objectives, keeping a daily reflection and progress log, and evaluating changes in your physical and mental well-being. These are all things that you can do. Embrace the trip with an open heart and mind, and may the chair yoga practice you engage in bring you the serenity, joy, and transformation you seek.

Chapter 12: Q&A and Troubleshooting

Common Challenges in Chair Yoga Practice

By practicing chair yoga, which is a wonderful way to enjoy the benefits of yoga practice, people of all ages and abilities are able to take use of the benefits that yoga has to offer. On the other hand, just like any other form of physical activity or pursuit of wellness, it comes with its own particular set of challenges that set it apart from other possibilities. In the following chapter, we will talk about some of the most common difficulties that people who practice chair yoga could have, and we will also present some suggestions to help them overcome these difficulties.

1. A limited range of motion available to the user

The restricted range of motion that can be brought on by a variety of situations, including but not limited to age, injury, or handicap, which is one of the most important challenges involved with chair yoga, is one of the most serious issues associated with chair yoga. On the other hand, there are certain individuals who, as a result of stiffness or discomfort in their joints, may find it difficult to achieve particular positions.

The idea is to adjust the postures so that they are suitable for each individual according to their needs. It is essential that you make use of a variety of props when it comes to stretching. Some examples of these props include yoga blocks and straps. Put your focus on moving in a relaxed manner, which will help you progressively build your flexibility over the course of several exercises. To emphasize how vital it is to pay attention to what your body is trying to tell you and to never go beyond what is comfortable for you, stress the importance of this.

2. Worries Regarding the Existence of a Balance

The capacity to maintain one's equilibrium can be challenging to accomplish, particularly for individuals who are of advanced age or who have mobility limitations. There is a possibility that the participants' fear of falling will hinder them from participating in yoga practice to its fullest extent.

The answer is to start with seated positions that provide support and stability because this is the solution. With the goal of gradually improving your stability and self-assurance, you should think about incorporating exercises that require you to maintain your balance while seated. It is possible to utilize the chair as a prop to offer support while you are performing standing poses. As your balance improves, you will be able to gradually minimize the amount of reliance you have on the chair.

3. An anxiety about being hurt

There is a possibility that some individuals are hesitant to begin practicing yoga because they are concerned about the possibility of exacerbating existing conditions or developing new injuries with the practice. It is probable that this fear is the result of a lack of understanding regarding the appropriate approach and alignment according to the subject matter.

A remedy to this problem is to educate participants on proper body mechanics and alignment in order to reduce the possibility that they may sustain an injury. It is of the utmost importance to lay a strong emphasis on the significance of training and listening to one's body while working within one's own bounds. When it comes to facilitating open communication and providing accommodations for individuals who have special injuries or conditions, encouraging open communication is a great way to work.

Number Four of the Accessibility Restrictions

People who reside in rural areas or those who have mobility issues and are unable to easily go to a studio may have limited access to chair yoga programs. This is because it is conceivable that these individuals will be unable to easily enter the studio.

It is possible to reach a broader audience by offering chair yoga classes that are delivered remotely via the use of video conferencing devices. This is the solution. It would be beneficial to make taped sessions available to folks so that they can practice whenever it is most conveniently for them. It is recommended that individuals who have limited mobility take into consideration the possibility of creating relationships with community organizations, senior centers, or healthcare facilities in order to offer seat yoga classes on the premises.

Addressing Physical Limitations

In spite of the fact that physical limitations may provide significant challenges when it comes to the practice of yoga, it is not necessary for these limitations to be impediments that hinder participation. The following are some of the ways that physical restrictions can be overcome via the practice of chair yoga:

Changes and alterations Adapted to the Specific Needs of You

Engage in one-on-one collaboration with participants in order to ascertain the specific limitations they are subject to and to create modifications that are tailored to fit their specific requirements. Depending on the circumstances, this may involve adjusting poses, making use of props, or focusing on other motions that produce results that are equal to those accomplished by the original action.

2. An Emphasis on Breathing and Maintaining Awareness of the Present Moment

By placing a larger emphasis on activities such as breathing exercises and mindfulness practices, it is possible to make these activities more accessible to those who have a wide range of physical abilities. It is important that participants be taught to focus their attention on the breath as a technique of fostering presence and awareness within the context of their practice.

A Method That Is Considered to Be Progressive

It is recommended that the practice of yoga be approached in a manner that is progressive, beginning with fundamental poses and gradually incorporating motions that are progressively more challenging as the practitioners build their strength, flexibility, and self-assurance within the practice. In order to make challenging poses more approachable, it is possible to break them down into smaller steps that are more manageable.

4. Support and Words of Encouragement Put in place an environment that is warm and welcoming, one that is inclusive, and one in which participants are encouraged to deepen their practice without feeling forced or evaluated in any manner. It is important to recognize and appreciate their achievements, regardless of how minor they may appear to be, and to provide them with positive reinforcement in order to boost their self-confidence and resolve.

Overcoming Mental Barriers to Yoga Practice

It is possible for individuals to face mental obstacles in addition to physical barriers, which prevent them from fully engaging in the practice of yoga to the extent that they are capable of doing so. The following is a list of mentally challenging situations that frequently arise, along with some strategies for conquering them:

(1) Confidence in Oneself

A significant number of individuals have emotions of self-doubt when they first start a new yoga practice. In particular, this is the case if individuals are frightened by the seeming difficulty of particular poses or by their own physical limitations.

In order to successfully implement the technique that needs you to provide a supportive and non-judgmental setting in which participants feel safe to explore and experiment with their practice, you will need to create an environment. They should be reminded that yoga is a journey, not a destination, and they should be encouraged to focus on making progress rather than obtaining perfection in their yoga practice.

The Fear of Failing to Accomplish It

Because of the fear of failing, some people may be dissuaded from attempting new things or pushing themselves outside of their comfort zone when it comes to yoga practice. This anxiety may contribute to the discouragement of individuals.

It is important to emphasize the idea that there is no such thing as failure in yoga; rather, there are only learning experiences that might occur. Participants should be encouraged to approach their practice with an attitude of openness and inquiry, letting go of whatever expectations they may have with regard to the practice, and receiving whatever comes their way.

3. Contrast and contrast together

Comparing oneself to other students in the class or to photographs of more experienced practitioners that are posted on social media can be detrimental to one's self-esteem and confidence. This is especially true when the comparison is negative.

Strategy: Remind the participants that yoga is a personal practice and that the way in which each person achieves their goals is different from the path that others pursue. It is important to encourage them to focus on their own personal development and to acknowledge and appreciate the many different skills and characteristics that they already possess.

not having enough patience

Some people may suffer feelings of frustration or discouragement if they do not see immediate effects from their yoga practice. This is because yoga is a discipline that is supposed to help people feel better.

Reminding people that transformation is a process that takes time and effort over a period of time is a vital step in the process of cultivating patience. It is important that you encourage them to continue their dedication to their practice and to have faith in the process, despite the fact that the progress may appear to be gradual or incremental.

Through addressing the common issues that are connected with chair yoga and providing solutions for overcoming those challenges, we may contribute to making chair yoga more accessible and enjoyable for people of all ages and abilities. Keeping in mind that yoga is ultimately about self-acceptance and self-discovery, and that the route that each individual travels is distinct, is an important thing to keep in mind. If we have patience, perseverance, and compassion for the people we are helping, we will be able to assist them in overcoming hurdles and experience the life-changing benefits that yoga practice may provide.

Conclusion

As we near the completion of our voyage through "28 Day Chair Yoga For Seniors," it is necessary to take a minute to reflect the transformational possibilities of the practices that we have studied and the adventure that we have set out on together. We have been exploring the peaceful yet profound world of chair yoga for the past month and a half. Chair yoga is a practice that is performed in a chair. It has come to our attention that chair yoga has the potential to act as a catalyst for better health, energy, and mental tranquility, regardless of the individual's age or physical limitations.

The purpose of this book is to cater to the special needs of senior citizens, and throughout its whole, we have explored a wide variety of topics with the objective of doing so. Methods such as guided meditations, mindful breathing exercises, mild stretches, and writing prompts for introspective reflection are included in this category. With each passing day, we are growing closer and closer to discovering the full potential of our bodies and minds, and we are learning to appreciate the beauty that can be found in movement, breath, and quiet. This is a process that is taking place.

The most important thing that we will take away from this trip is the realization that yoga is so much more than just a series of physical positions. Yoga is a discipline that encompasses all aspects of mental, physical, and spiritual well-being. It is at this moment in our trip that we have reached the most significant realization. Having developed a more profound awareness and compassion for ourselves, we have acquired the ability to pay attention to the direction that our bodies provide and to respect their inherent capacity for healing. This ability has allowed us to develop the ability to heal ourselves. The practice of yoga, as we have come to understand it, is not about obtaining perfection or reaching some arbitrary target; rather, it is about showing up exactly as we are and discovering calm in the here and now.

The other side of the coin is that we have built a sense of camaraderie and support that has assisted us in getting through even the most challenging of days. This is probably even more important than you might think. Throughout the course of this road that we have taken together, we have been reminded on numerous occasions that we are not the only ones suffering through the difficulties that we are. It has been brought to our attention that there is power in solidarity, and that there is strength in the experience that is shared by others. We are able to take the first step into the mat each day with the assurance that we are supported at every level of the process because of the encouragement that we receive from our fellow seniors. This gives us the confidence to take the first step onto the mat.

I would want to express my gratitude for the opportunity to be of assistance to you throughout this 28 days of chair yoga practice. When I think back on the commitment that I made to you at the beginning of our journey, I am overcome with feelings of appreciation. My intention was to provide you with a road map that would lead you to improved vitality, resilience, and positive experiences; to make available to you the resources and information that you require in order to reclaim control over your health and well-being; to make these things available to you. And now that we are nearing to the finish of our time together, I am positive that we have managed to fulfill that commitment.

On the other hand, there is one thing that I hope you will take away from this book, and that is the awareness that you are capable of a great deal more than you currently believe you are capable of. Regardless of your age or the status of your physical health, you have the potential to make changes to your life and to embrace each moment with open arms. This is something that you possess within yourself. You will realize that you have acquired a renewed feeling of joy and purpose as you progress through the process of cultivating a consistent yoga practice. This will allow you to tap the limitless reservoir of strength, tranquility, and energy that is already present inside you.

I want to encourage you to take the information you've received and the habits you've developed with you when you turn the final page of this book and prepare to return to the real world. This is because of the reasons stated above. Always remember to make time for yourself on a daily basis, paying attention to the needs of your body and working to cultivate the calmness of your mind. Remember that you are never going through this journey alone yourself; your fellow seniors are there to encourage you and cheer you on at every single stage of the road. Keep this in mind at all times.

I want to express my appreciation for the fact that you have chosen to take part in this chair yoga practice with me for a period of 28 days and have provided me with the opportunity to guide you through it. It is my sincere appreciation that you have given me the chance to be a part of the transformation that you are undergoing. Being able to go beside you on this incredible journey has been a privilege and a source of great pleasure. You will continue to be a shining example of the limitless potential that is inside you, and your brilliance will continue to shine brilliantly. Namaste.